To Ann & Dwight,
From Mom D.

Alice and I were greatly
blessed by this book.
Mom D.

FRUCTOSE EXPOSED

The Sweet Truth About America's
Expanding Waistline And Failing Health

October 27, 2010

Lyons

FRUCTOSE EXPOSED

The Sweet Truth About America's Expanding Waistline And Failing Health

M. Frank Lyons II, M.D.

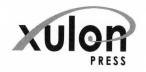

Fructose Exposed
The Sweet Truth About America's Expanding Waistline
And Failing Health
by M. Frank Lyons II, M.D.

Printed in the United States of America

ISBN 9781612150253

www.xulonpress.com

Dedication

This book is dedicated to the individuals who struggle daily with diabetes, high blood pressure, fatty liver disease, heart disease, obesity, kidney damage, cancers, and other disorders because of a lack of understanding of the destruction that excess fructose is creating in their bodies.

Acknowledgements

I would like to thank my patients for tolerating my continued bombardment of the detriment of the Western diet on their health. They have endured my many discussions concerning lessons in biochemistry, metabolism, and pathophysiology of fats and carbohydrates.

Many thanks and deepest gratitude goes out to my sister, Deborah Shucka, for the editing, providing emotional support, and assisting me during manuscript preparation. She has taught me so much about writing over the years, and she is an outstanding critic as only a big sister can be.

Others that helped in the review process of this text include: Dr. Michael Kimmey, Maggie Steenrod, Bob Steenrod, Mark Lyons, Allisyn Deyo-Martin, and Dr. Brian Mulhall. I am most appreciative of their instructive criticism and assistance in the preparation of the book.

Pertinent to this planet, I am most grateful to my spouse, Clare, for tolerating my many hours of researching, typing, discussing, and editing. Without her daily support this book would not have reached its present form.

Finally, not of this world; I want to thank my God from above for giving me the ability to transcribe these vitally important messages about fructose into readable form for my patients and others interested in improving their health.

"Everything in Excess is Opposed to Nature."
Hippocrates

Table of Contents

"Apply thy heart unto instruction, and thine ears to the words of knowledge." *Proverbs 23:12*

Introduction

꙳

In May of 2010 the White House Task Force on Childhood Obesity released their report to the President of the United States. This 120 page document was amazing in its depth and breadth of recommendations for the federal, state, and local governments to initiate numerous programs in order to solve the obesity problem that plagues the youth of America. As I read through this lengthy manuscript (fortunately not as long as the health care bill that was passed just two months earlier into law but not read by our elected officials), I was struck by the lack of science as it relates to metabolism, nutrition needs and diets destructive to the health of the human body.

When guidelines are placed before an audience, they should be understood by all who read them. More importantly, the readership should understand why the guidelines are important for the reader to follow—otherwise, the guidelines will fall on deaf ears. Nothing is accomplished. A recent article in the *Archives of Internal Medicine* revealed that, in spite of intensive weight loss counseling by health care providers, children did not lose weight in the follow-up period. Yet one of the recommendations of the Task Force report is to mandate the initiation of a similar counseling and education program.

In order to make an impact on poor health we must first educate ourselves about the causes of poor health. We should not just focus on a government fix to the problem, especially when the recommendation is not totally accurate. A great example of this was the revised U.S. Department of Agriculture (USDA) "Food Pyramid" that was released to the American public in 2005. For 35 years the previous pyramid had not been nutritionally sound; yet, we had been following the poor dietary advice outlined in the "Food Pyramid" from the federal government.

Likewise, they now want to restrict the salt content in food in an attempt to lower the blood pressure of Americans. High blood pressure is the most common, treatable medical condition in the United States at the present time. By the time you finish reading this book, you will understand, and rightfully conclude, that salt is not the initiating problem for high blood pressure. Rather, it is the daily consumption of excess fructose that leads to salt retention. The high blood pressure follows from the salt retention. Removing the salt does not reverse the continued salt retention caused by the sustained intemperate indulgence of fructose— that requires reduction in daily fructose consumption. More on that in my "task force" recommendations near the end of this book.

First, I must take you through some important background information about the problems related to fructose. If you understand what fructose is, where it is found in your diet, and what your body does with excess fructose, you will be better armed with the knowledge that will motivate you to improve your diet. Those nutritional changes implemented by you will lead to improved health, less need for medications, laboratory testing, doctor's office visits, and lost time from work. All the while, you and I will not need a whole new set of government mandates. We will know why and how to make better choices at the supermarket, restaurant, and dinner table.

If we follow some of the dietary guidelines prescribed by the White House Task Force, we consume excess fructose. This simple one day menu makes the point:

Breakfast:
  1 cup Rice Krispies cereal/1 tsp. sugar (2.1 grams)
  1 cup orange juice (11.1 grams)
  1 cup of 2% milk (0 grams)
  1 slice multigrain toast/1 Tbs. jam (4.6 grams)
    Total: 17.8 grams fructose

Lunch:
  2 sl. wheat bread, peanut butter, jelly (6.9 grams)
  1 medium apple (12.6 grams)
  1 fruit juice box (17 grams)
  1 serving of carrot sticks (1.7 grams)
    Total: 38.2 grams fructose

Afterschool Snack:
  1 orange and 1 oatmeal raisin cookie (12 grams)
  1 cup 2% milk (0 grams)
    Total: 12 grams fructose

Dinner:
  Chicken breast (0 grams)
  1 cup brown rice (0.3 grams)
  1 cup cauliflower in cheese sauce (1 gram)
  1 cup milk (0 grams)
  1 cup salad/ranch dressing (1.1 grams)
    Total: 2.4 grams fructose

Evening Snack:
  ½ cup low fat ice cream (8.2 grams)
    Total: 8.2 grams fructose

Daily Total: 78.6 grams fructose

You will note from this diet plan that they drank no soda pop. This is atypical, especially among male youth in America. If you added a bottle of Gatorade and a 12 ounce can of cola to the menu, which would provide another 36 grams of fructose for the day for a total of 114.6 grams. Another thing I tried to do was to include two servings of fresh fruit and at least three servings of vegetables/whole grains for the day. I also tried to minimize "fast foods," sugar-sweetened snack foods and high fat foods. These are all recommendations that are found in the Task Force report. While I did give the child a small glass of orange juice for breakfast and a box of juice for lunch, it is often difficult to stay away from all forms of juice in kids' diets. This is a convenience as much as anything. The Task Force report recommends fruit smoothies; however, these drinks are loaded with large quantities of fructose. Many shopping malls in large metropolitan areas today contain several fruit smoothie restaurant chains, and our youth flock to them as the smoothie is touted as a healthy, natural snack alternative to soda pop.

The human body was never designed to properly metabolize 78.6 grams of fructose daily, let alone 114.6 grams. Our liver was constructed in a way that we can only process around 15 grams per day without leading to destructive biochemical reactions that affect the rest of the body. The remainder must go somewhere. Science is now shedding light on the metabolic outcome of chronic excess fructose ingestion. This book will enlighten you about that science.

I showed the above diet to a colleague of mine who has three teenagers. She informed me that her teenagers consume far more sugared foods and larger portions than I listed in my simple menu. Additionally, they will consume many more snacks in a day than I included. Interestingly, none of them are presently overweight. As you will learn though, their metabolism may be messed up in spite of their lack of obesity. This point is just as significant.

As you can see from my example, if you follow the new USDA "Food Pyramid" guidelines, reduce salt in your diet, follow a low-fat diet and avoid "fast food" dining, you will make no significant impact on the quantity of fructose consumed. By the end of this book I hope you will hopefully have a better understanding of the dilemma we all face at the supermarket, the shopping mall, the "fast food" restaurant and at the dining room table.

The other major aspect of this book is the discussion about the science that surrounds the medical disorders that develop because of chronic, excess ingestion of fructose. This information is reviewed so that you will understand the damage you are causing by going down this deadly nutrition highway. You will learn how many of these problems can not only be prevented, but can also be reversed once you undertake major changes in your diet. This is especially true for the younger generations that are already suffering from metabolic changes which will lead to long-term medical disasters if not arrested. If caught early in life, they are reversible with massive reduction in fructose intake, not salt avoidance or other "Food Pyramid" guidelines. Government intervention is not the answer. **Daily reduction in fructose consumption is the key to better health for all of us.**

Pearls

- The primary cause of obesity and altered metabolism of the youth and adults of America is chronic, excess fructose intake.
- Personal changes in your diet, not government intervention, are the keys to reversing the destructive processes of present USDA dietary guidelines.

"All men make mistakes, but only wise men learn from their mistakes." *Winston Churchill*

Chapter 1

The American Diet Gone Awry

"**D**ad, why is high fructose corn syrup absolutely terrible for us?" One of my daughters had just read a story on the Internet warning people about its impact on health.

It was with that prompting that I challenged myself to see if I could figure out whether her story was correct; and if so, why. Why would high fructose corn syrup be so bad for our health? Was there something unique about this manufactured sugar that was worse than table sugar?

I had just completed writing a book concerning the deplorable state of health in America due to the imbalance of fat in the Western diet (*42 Days to a New Life: The Importance of a Balanced Fat Intake That Will Change Your Health [From Alpha to Omega]*, Xulon Press, 2007). Mountains of research I unearthed in the medical literature revealed that our diet has caused numerous medical conditions that should not be seen, or should occur at far less frequencies, than occur in America. I also learned that the manufactured food industry, the Department of Agriculture and the federal government have done little to reverse the damage created by our diet.

Let me explain. Trans fats were introduced into the Western diet in 1911. It was not until after World War II

21

that consumption of these deadly fats began to take off in America. By 1958 it was clear that trans fats were the major contributor to heart disease and cancer in the United States.

Doctor Ancel Keys, an internationally known nutrition professor at the University of Minnesota, was commissioned by the U.S. government in the 1950s to determine the cause of the rapidly-rising incidence of heart disease and cancer that was occurring at alarming rates all across America. After exhaustive data analysis, he determined that the primary cause of these conditions was the human consumption of trans fats in the Western diet. He warned the Food and Drug Administration in 1958 that these manufactured fats should be eliminated from our diet. This has still not been accomplished. And, sadly enough, many Americans continue to suffer from heart attacks, sudden death, strokes, cancer and many other inflammatory diseases because of continued consumption of trans fats.

Additionally, there are two essential fats (omega-3 fatty acids and omega-6 fatty acids) necessary to maintain health in the human body. We do not have the metabolic machinery to make these fats so we must consume them daily or suffer the consequences from their deficiencies. Our major sources of omega-3 fatty acids were eliminated from the American diet in the 1960s when the Food and Drug Administration removed cod liver oil from the diet and mandated the pasteurization of all milk distributed in the United States. Cattle feed was converted from a diet rich in omega-3 fatty acids (grass and grains) to omega-6 fatty acids (corn silage and soybean meal). This converted the meat and milk of these animals from being a rich source of omega-3 fatty acids to omega-6 rich fat.

We are what we eat. The importance of this conversion in the diet of the dairy cows was that omega-3 fatty-acid-rich food (grass and grains) reduces inflammatory diseases, heart disease and cancer. Diets rich in omega-6 fatty acids do just the opposite. Corn and soybeans have never been a natural diet of dairy cattle. This change in their diet, and the pasteurization of their milk (which destroys the omega-3 fatty acids found in the milk), has been one of the most catastrophic experiments in nutrition in world history. **As goes the American diet, so goes the rest of the modern world.** Many countries have fallen prey to the ill effects of trans fats as they have adopted our diet of "fast foods" and processed foods containing trans fats.

The use of trans fats, the drastic reduction in the consumption of omega-3 fatty acids, and the significant increase in omega-6 fatty acid consumption in the American diet has led to an explosion of inflammatory diseases (explained in greater detail in my previous book), heart disease, cancer, and death (Table 1) that dwarfs natural catastrophes such as tsunamis, earthquakes, hurricanes, tornados and the like (Table 2).

Table 1. Deaths from Diseases in America in 2006

Heart Disease	631,636
Cancer	559,888
Stroke	137,119
Alzheimer's Disease	72,432

We see the devastating effects of numerous natural catastrophes every year. Many lives are lost because of these disasters (see Table 2); on the other hand, these dietary changes are all manmade. While the travesty of the damage suffered by an earthquake or hurricane is not reversible, the damage caused by our diet can be turned around or avoided altogether.

Table 2. Deaths from Natural Catastrophes

Chili Earthquake Feb. 2010	1,600
Haiti Earthquake Jan. 2010	222,570
Hurricane Katrina Aug. 2005	1,836
Sumatra Earthquake Dec. 2004	227,898
25 Worst U.S. Tornadoes **1880–Present**	3,755
Deaths from All Earthquakes in 2009	1,783

Not all deaths from the major diseases (Table 1) are solely due to the changes in the makeup of fat that occurred in the Western diet over the last hundred years. We have seen however, that the elimination of trans fats will drastically lower deaths due to heart disease. Finland removed trans fats from their diet in the 1970s, and heart disease decreased by 50% over the next quarter century. While there is no good data for total lives saved, it is clear that many people would live much healthier lives if our diet returned to that seen before World War II.

It has become clear to me that the health of our bodies benefits when we consume animal products and animals that forage on a natural diet of grasses and grains. It is only when we try to improve on nature by altering animal feed (for reasons of cost containment and mass production) that we produce food substances that are not natural to our metabolism, health and ultimately, to our survival. Converting a cow's meat (and milk) being fed an unnatural diet rich in omega-6 foods (corn silage, soybean meal, etc.) back to an omega-3 rich diet (grasses, grains) would have a huge impact on the health of America. Additionally, producing milk that is processed in a way that preserves the integrity of the omega-3 fatty acids, rather than a 19th century cleansing technique developed by Dr. Louis Pasteur that destroys the integrity of omega-3 fatty acids, seems paramount.

Developing alternative technologies for food production, food preservation and animal diets in the 21st century should be a high priority. Additionally, methods need to be developed to improve the quality of our milk and animal meats, rather than just going from pasteurization to ultra pasteurization to preserve milk, or continuing to produce meats that are rich in inflammatory omega-6 fats. Ultra pasteurization only further denatures any omega-3 fatty acid that may have survived pasteurization at a lower temperature. And, returning farm animals to a diet rich in grass-, flax-, grain- and algae-based feeds would dramatically improve human health in short order.

Likewise, the trans fat story is just as tragic. Trans fats are a family of manufactured omega-6 fatty acids produced from vegetable oils. These fats were initially developed in Germany as a lubricant for machinery. As the properties of these fats became better understood, they were found to preserve food and prevent spoilage by reducing oxidation of the natural fats found in foods. Oxidation is a natural process that causes fat to become rancid. The oxidation process is dramatically reduced with the addition of trans fats to processed food such as crackers, cookies, candies, cakes, ice cream, breads and pastries. It has been clear for over fifty years that these manufactured fats are a leading contributor to many of the leading killer diseases of America (Table 1). They continue to play an important role in the cause of numerous cancers, heart disease, inflammatory diseases, long-term suffering and premature death. Some counties (the counties of New York City, King County in Washington state, etc.) across the United States are now beginning to mandate the reduction of dietary consumption of these deadly fats in restaurants.

Unfortunately, these municipalities are following the same advice as the food labeling mandate of the federal government. The FDA states that so long as a serving size of trans fat is less than 500 mg per serving, the food label can say zero grams Trans fat per serving. Communities are following suit with similar guidelines. A serving must contain less than 500 mg of trans fat for the food to be labeled "Zero Grams Trans Fat." This 'fake labeling' seems to defeat the purpose of eliminating trans fats, as they are toxic to the human body in any quantity.

Total elimination of Trans fats from the food chain as seen in Finland would produce profound benefits on the health of this nation within just a few years.

Misleading the public with fallacious food-labeling practices, and government mandated artificial reduction of trans fats in menus of restaurants, does not improve your health. You need to become an educated consumer to make real changes that improve your health over the long term.

We need to learn the code words for Trans fats (hydrogenated and partially hydrogenated), and we must read the ingredient list of the food label. If it contains these fats put the product back on the shelf of the grocery store and choose an alternative product.

It was with this reflection that I began to realize the same story is being repeated with high fructose corn syrup (HFCS). As I will describe in more detail later, HFCS is a manufactured sugar derived from a food that was never meant to produce sugar for human consumption. The health ramifications of this deadly sugar are beginning to emerge all over the planet as high fructose corn syrup has now replaced sugar as the primary sweetening agent the world over. In the United States HFCS has increased from no consumption per person in 1970 to 44 pounds per person, per year by 2000.

Initially, my research led to an indictment of just this manufactured sugar. As I continued to unearth more information however, it became clear that high fructose corn syrup per se is not the sugar enemy of our health. Fructose, in general, no matter the source, is the true culprit. It does not matter whether the fructose is from table sugar, HFCS, purified fructose, fruits or fruit juices. **Fructose, in excess, alters the metabolism of the human body.** This change in the body's chemistry leads to devastating changes in our health. Fructose consumption has exploded throughout the world over the past half century. Because of this, we are now seeing the emergence of catastrophic effects on the health of people around the world in proportions unfathomable before.

As I take you through the history of sugar, high fructose corn syrup development, fructose consumption, and its now-recognized deadly effects, I hope you will begin to realize how important it is for you to take a close look at the fructose products you consume daily. The choices you make for you and your family will have life-long effects on your health, your quality of life as you age, and your longevity.

The questions raised by my daughter are certainly questions that many of you may be asking yourselves. My goal in writing this book is to answer those questions both for my daughter and for you, the reader.

Pearls

- Eliminate all trans fats (hydrogenated and partially hydrogenated vegetable oils) from your diet.
- Enrich your diet with omega-3 fatty acids.
- Reduce the omega-6 fatty acid content in your diet.
- Fructose, in excess, alters the metabolism of the human body.

> **"One should eat to live, not live to eat."**
> *Benjamin Franklin*

Chapter 2

We Are What We Eat!!

A sixteen-year-old male came to see me a few months ago. He was accompanied by his mother, who was rather distraught. The young man had previously seen a gastrointestinal specialist for abnormally elevated liver chemistries. After a vigorous evaluation that consisted of numerous blood tests, radiologic studies, and a liver biopsy, the specialist informed the adolescent that he suffered from a fatty liver. What was worse, the liver disease was quite advanced, and he would soon develop cirrhosis like that seen in alcoholics.

When they inquired as to a treatment, the patient was instructed to lose weight, but there was no specific therapy. His weight was 265 pounds, which is significantly increased, even for the six foot, two inch frame of this young man. He was also suffering from high blood pressure, high cholesterol, elevated triglycerides (another type of blood fat) and borderline diabetes.

The mom was not satisfied with what she was hearing, so she sought a second opinion from the University of Washington Hospital in Seattle. Again, the mother and her son heard the same advice. They returned to their family physician seeking further recommendations. They were referred to me as I have had some success in treating patients who suffer from fatty liver disease over the past ten years.

I questioned the young man about his diet. As is true of many teenagers in America today, he frequently consumed fast foods. He also drank at least three to four cans or bottles of sugared, non-diet sodas daily.

I had learned from previous research concerning fatty liver that many of the deleterious effects of this potentially deadly disorder can be reversed with the elimination of trans fats and the consumption of omega-3 fatty acids on a regular basis. I also realized during my earlier investigations that some individuals, especially younger people who consume soda pop daily, did not respond to my treatment regimen very well. It wasn't until I began my homework for this book that I began to understand why. By the time you have finished reading this book, it will also be clear to you.

What is important to understand is that nearly all of the popular brands of soda pop contain only high fructose corn syrup as their sugar sweetener. This was not true as recently as twenty-five years ago. Many processed food manufacturers have replaced table sugar with high fructose corn syrup. When I began my exploration into the ill effects of high fructose corn syrup, I jumped to the conclusion that, in addition to his dietary indiscretion of excess trans fat intake and the lack of omega-3 fatty acids in his diet, this manufactured sugar was a major cause of the liver damage and other metabolic problems of this adolescent.

I informed the patient and his mother that if he did not take drastic steps immediately to reverse the liver damage, he would develop cirrhosis within the next decade of his life. I instructed them to eliminate all trans fats, incorporate omega-3 fatty acids into the diet two to three times per day, and to eliminate all high fructose corn syrup from his diet. He and his mother have taken my advice to heart. He has made major changes in his diet, and he is exercising more regularly. His liver chemistries have begun to normalize, and his weight is beginning to fall. Incidentally, he also feels much healthier than he has felt in many years.

Why eliminate high fructose corn syrup? What I learned from my fatty liver patients who did not respond to my treatment regimen (elimination of trans fats, addition of omega-3 fatty acids, and reduction of omega-6 fatty acids) was that they were all heavy consumers of this sugar. If they would comply with removal of this manufactured sugar from their diet, their livers would soon be the benefactors of the healing process that my other patients (without significant consumption of high fructose corn syrup) with fatty liver have seen.

What is the problem with high fructose corn syrup? As this book unfolds, I will try to make it clear that this sugar and other sources of fructose not only cause fatty liver, but continued ingestion will lead to a multiplicity of disorders that are now developing all over the planet in younger and younger individuals. Fatty liver is just the tip of the iceberg.

As I described in this young man's medical history, he also suffers from other health issues. He has high blood pressure, elevated blood levels of cholesterol and triglycerides and borderline diabetes. As I will elaborate individually in subsequent chapters, you will see that all of these medical conditions have now been attributed to regular consumption of high fructose corn syrup and other fructose-containing foods and beverages. This latter point was a shock to me when I first uncovered research data that incriminates not just high fructose corn syrup, but fructose from any source.

After you have completed reading this book, hopefully you too will take this warning seriously. More importantly, you will also understand why high fructose intake should be eliminated from all diets. While my initial conclusion caused me to convict high fructose corn syrup as "the evil sugar" of our time, continued research convinced me that any sugar or food source containing fructose consumed in excess quantities on a daily basis leads to the same disease processes. Whether we consume excess table sugar, fruit, fruit juices, honey or high fructose corn syrup does not matter. Excess consumption of fructose from any source leads to the devastating effects on our health that I outline in future chapters.

I have further counseled my patient that he needs to drastically reduce all forms of fructose from his diet. He is now taking an active role in grocery shopping with his mom. They are working together to reverse his liver disease, lower his blood levels of cholesterol and triglycerides, and keep his blood sugars in good control through elimination of most sources of fructose that used to be a regular part of his daily eating habits.

As you process the information that follows, perhaps you can apply this knowledge toward your own diet. Just as the young man I discussed at the outset of this chapter is beginning to correct the ill effects of fructose on his health, you might also be able to produce long-lasting health benefits for yourself.

You must first learn what fructose is, where it is found in your diet, how it is processed in your body and what happens if you chronically consume too much of it.

Pearls

- **Excess fructose in our diet is the cause of many of the health issues that have emerged in America over the past three decades.**

"It is health that is real wealth and not pieces of gold and silver." *Mohandas Gandhi*

Chapter 3

Fundamentals of Nutrition

E ntire college lecture courses with accompanying text books are taught concerning human nutrition. My goal in this chapter is to condense that information and give you a brief overview of the nutritional needs for the maintenance of health. Nutritional imbalance can cause serious consequences to our bodies. Lack of essential nutrients can cause many diseases and even death. Likewise, an excess of some nutrients can lead to many disorders and fatality. Balance is the key. Finding this balance requires an understanding of what are essential nutrients. Beyond this we must have a grasp of the amounts of required consumption on a regular basis, and the consequences of consuming deficient, or excess quantities, of these indispensable nutrients.

The first fundamental message of understanding nutrition is that there are certain basic nutrients we must consume regularly because our body cannot manufacture them. These include: water, vitamins, minerals, protein, and fat (Table 1). Without these basic substances in our diet, we suffer from malnutrition, illnesses and premature death.

Table 1. Essential Nutrients That Must Be Ingested

Water	Any form
Vitamins	A (Retinol), B1 (Thiamine), B2 (Riboflavin), B3 (Niacin), B5 (Pantothenic Acid), B6 (Pyridoxine), B7 (Biotin), B9 (Folic Acid), B-12 (Cobalamin), C (Ascorbic acid), D (Ergocalciferol), E (Alpha-Tocopherol), K (Phylloquinone). Choline is considered to be an essential vitamin by some nutrition experts; however the body does manufacture this vitamin.
Minerals	Sodium, Chlorine (chloride), Potassium, Calcium, Phosphorus, Magnesium, Iron, Zinc, Iodine, Selenium, Copper, Manganese, Fluorine (fluoride), Chromium, Molybdenum
Protein (Essential Amino Acids)	Histidine, Isoleucine, Leucine, Lysine, Methionine, Phenylalanine, Threonine, Tryptophan, Valine. (There are 11 nonessential amino acids that can be manufactured by the body with adequate nutrition.)
Fat	Omega-3 Fatty Acids (Alpha Linolenic Acid [ALA, the parent oil], Eicosapentanoic acid [EPA], Docosahexanoic Acid [DHA]), Omega-6 Fatty Acid (Linoleic Acid)

The human body will not remain healthy, and in many instances not even survive, without consuming these necessary components on a recurring basis.

Numerous diseases develop if we do not consume essential nutrients on a regular schedule as our bodies cannot maintain daily metabolic needs (Table 2).

An amazing documentation of an essential nutrient deficiency which led to catastrophe was documented in the journals recording the circumnavigation of the world by

Table 2. Diseases of Essential Nutrient Deficiencies

Essential Nutrient	Disease	Time to Disease State
Water	Dehydration, Death	days – wks.
Vitamin A	Night Blindness, Death	mos. – yrs.
Thiamine (B1)	Heart Failure, Wasting	wks. – mos.
Riboflavin (B2)	Rash, Photophobia, Mouth Cracks	wks. – mos.
Niacin (B3)	Diarrhea, Painful Tongue	wks. – mos.
Pantothenic Acid (B5)	Vomiting, Fatigue, Hypoglycemia	wks. – mos.
Pyridoxime (B6)	Anemia, Depression, Rash	wks. – mos.
Biotin (B7)	Depression, Rash, Heart Dz	wks. – mos.
Folic Acid (B9)	Anemia, Infection, Spina Bifida, Cleft Palate, Anencephaly	wks. – mos.

Cobalamin (B12)	Anemia, Neuropathy, Dementia	mos. – yrs.
Vitamin C	Anemia, Bleeding Gums, Death, Decreased Wound Healing	wks. – mos.
Vitamin D	Bone Dz, Muscle spasms, Increased Cancer Risk, Weight Gain, Depression	mos. – yrs.
Vitamin E	Anemia, Bleeding, Neuropathy	mos. – yrs.
Vitamin K	Bleeding, Bone Dz	mos. – yrs.
Sodium	Hypotension, Seizures, Death	days
Chloride	No Known Diet is Deficient	unknown
Potassium	Muscle Weakness, Confusion	days
Calcium	Bone Dz, Muscle Spasms, Stunted Growth	days
Phosphorus	Muscle Weakness, Bone Pain	days
Magnesium	Weakness, Confusion, Seizures	days
Iron	Anemia, Weakness, Confusion	wks. – mos.
Zinc	Growth Retardation, Hair Loss, Decreased Wound Healing	wks. – mos.
Iodine	Thyroid Dz, Mental Retardation	mos. – yrs.

Selenium	Heart Dz	mos. – yrs.
Copper	Anemia, Bone Dz	mos. – yrs.
Manganese	Poor Wound Healing, Bone Dz	mos. – yrs.
Fluoride	Tooth Decay	mos. – yrs.
Chromium	Abnormal Glucose Metabolism	mos. – yrs.
Molybdenum	None Observed in America	unknown
Protein	Muscle Wasting, Hair Loss, Death	mos. – yrs.
Omega-3 Fat	Inflammation, Cancer, Death	mos. – yrs.
Omega-6 Fat	Rash, Impotence, Death	mos. – yrs.

(Dz = disease, wks. = weeks, mos. = months, yrs. = years)

Ferdinand Magellan and his men. They departed the west coast of South America in late 1520 at its southern tip and traveled 96 days across the Pacific Ocean covering several thousand miles. During that three month crossing, Magellan lost over half of his ships' crew to scurvy (vitamin C deficiency) by the time they arrived in Guam. Only the sailors who consumed the rats on board the ship survived. Rats make their own vitamin C. The ingestion of vitamin C by consuming the rats was enough to allow the sailors to survive.

Likewise, an excess consumption of many of these essentials may also affect your health (Table 3). My previous book revealed the price our body pays for excess omega-6 fatty acid and trans fat ingestion. We develop numerous inflammatory diseases that lead to major suffering and premature death. Diseases such as arthritis, some cancers, heart attacks, depression and dementia are just some of those described in the book *"42 Days to a New Life."* I would encourage you to read it as a supplement to what is outlined in this text.

One of the fascinating stories of excess ingestion of a single essential nutrient is that of the men who participated in the Lewis and Clark Expedition. They had to hunt the food they consumed during the two year journey. These men consumed upwards of twenty pounds of meat (protein) per day. The fascinating aspect of what would be considered gluttony to most of us today is that all of these men lived into their 80s (no death due to premature heart disease). We now know that the grass-fed animals (buffalo, deer, elk, antelope, etc.) that they consumed do not cause heart disease, cancer and other inflammatory diseases we see today with the Western diet. Our present diet contains products of corn-fed (inflammatory omega-6 fat) animals and processed foods filled with manufactured **trans** fats.

Table 3. Diseases of Essential Nutrient Excesses

Nutrient	Diseases
Water	Diabetes Insipidus (water intoxication)
Vitamin A	Liver Dz, Diarrhea, Bone Pain, Rash, Hair Loss
Thiamine (B1)	No Toxicity Known
Riboflavin (B2)	Sore Throat, Sore Red Tongue
Niacin (B3)	Nausea, Vomiting, Rash, Liver Dz
Pantothenic Acid (B5)	Water Retention
Pyridoxine (B6)	Bloating, Depression, Nerve Damage, Rash
Biotin (B7)	No Toxicity Known
Folic Acid (B9)	Masks Vitamin B12 Deficiency
Cobalamin	No Toxicity Known
Vitamin C	Diarrhea, Kidney Stones, Fatigue, Insomnia

Vitamin D	High Calcium, Body Damage, Headache, Nausea
Vitamin E	Fatigue, Nausea, Heart Failure, Death
Vitamin K	No Known Toxicity
Sodium	Hypertension, Water Retention
Chloride	No Known Toxicity
Potassium	Muscle Weakness, Vomiting
Calcium	Constipation, Kidney Stones
Phosphorus	Tissue Calcification
Magnesium	Diarrhea, Muscle Cramps
Iron	Abdominal Pain, Fatigue, Liver Dz, Joint Pain
Zinc	Nausea, Vomiting, Diarrhea, Headache
Iodine	Thyroid Enlargement, Low Thyroid Function
Selenium	Nausea, Abdominal Pain, Nerve and Liver Dz
Copper	Vomiting, Diarrhea, Liver Dz
Fluoride	Nausea, Vomiting, Tooth Damage, Diarrhea
Chromium	Skin Eruptions
Protein	May Accelerate Known Kidney Dz, Obesity
Omega-3 Fatty Acid	No Known Toxicity, Obesity (excess calories)
Omega-6 Fatty Acid	Inflammatory Disease, Obesity (excess calories)

Dz = Disease

If we consume several glasses of water per day, take a multivitamin (or consume foods or other supplements that provide these essential nutrients), consume four to six ounces of high quality protein and supplement our diet with essential fatty acids (fish oil, flax oil, etc) we could maintain our health as long as we were consuming enough total calories to meet our energy requirements. Additionally, if we reduce the excess omega-6 fatty acids, fructose and a glut of calories from many food sources, we would appreciate an improvement in our health.

Several factors play into meeting energy requirements on a daily basis. Your age, activity level, the presence of underlying chronic medical conditions, and immediate illnesses or injuries all demand varying amounts of energy intake to heal and maintain the human condition. Energy intake is measured in calories. A typical adult needs to consume between 1500 calories (for an older, healthy woman with a sedentary lifestyle) and 3000 calories or more (for a young, adult male with an active lifestyle).

When we consume fewer calories than are needed to meet our energy requirements, we lose weight at the expense of burning excess stored fat. Additionally, if we consume excess calories we convert the extra calories into fat, and we begin to gain weight. Energy requirements decline with age and decreased activity. In addition, men need more calories to maintain a larger muscle mass than women.

You will notice that carbohydrates are missing from the list of necessary nutrients of regular dietary consumption. The next chapter will discuss carbohydrates in depth; however, it is important to understand that carbohydrates are not on the "essential" list of nutrients for nearly all human beings. There is a very rare disorder seen in children that requires glucose to be consumed to maintain normal body function. The rest of us are spared this genetic deficiency and do not need to eat carbohydrates in order to maintain our health.

Presently, Americans consume approximately 40-50% of their energy needs through the intake of various carbohydrates. The U.S. Department of Agriculture's (USDA)

"Food Pyramid" recommended a diet rich in carbohydrates to the U.S. consumer in the 1970s that included 6-11 servings of breads/cereals, 2-4 servings of fruits, and 3-5 servings of vegetables per day. While that was revised in 2005, the USDA's "New Food Pyramid" still recommends 16-20 servings of carbohydrates per day. It is unclear to me why the USDA would increase recommendations for even more carbohydrates as we now realize the reason America is becoming obese is because of massive, excessive consumption of carbohydrates. While carbohydrates clearly meet our energy needs, excess carbohydrate ingestion (fructose in particular) is the cause of numerous weight and health issues in America. Additionally, fats and proteins also meet "essential" nutrient needs as well as energy needs. If taken to excess, fat and protein consumption will also lead to obesity and health issues. But, the human gastrointestinal system signals our brain much more effectively to stop eating when fats and protein are the initiator of that signal rather than fructose-based carbohydrates. Most people actually keep their weight under control or lose weight if they avoid carbohydrates, especially fructose-containing foods and beverages. Numerous studies have validated this point; however, the USDA continues to warn the American public against daily ingestion of a low carbohydrate, high protein and high fat diet.

Numerous, well-controlled research studies reveal that diets rich in carbohydrates and low in fat cause an increased illness and death rate over time compared to high protein, moderated fat and low carbohydrate diets. A recent three arm study published in the New England Journal of Medicine compared the "Atkins" type diet, the USDA-style high carbohydrate, low fat diet and the "Mediterranean" diet over a long period of time. The study revealed the best sustained weight loss, decreased morbidity and mortality in all categories occurred in the subjects who consumed the "Atkins" type, high protein, moderate fat, low carbohydrate diet.

The federal government and agribusiness continually make cholesterol and saturated fat ingestion the enemy of our bodies. As I pointed out in *42 Days to a New Life*, the culprit of fat ingestion is consumption of "manufactured" vegetable **trans** fats and an imbalance of omega-3 and omega-6 fatty acids in our diet. Plant oils such as cottonseed and soybean oil are subjected to heat and pressure to alter their chemical structure. As this occurs, it changes the character of the oil into a grease-like state (Crisco, etc.) that prevents food from becoming rancid and spoiling in a normal fashion. Think about a Twinkie. It can sit on the store shelf for years without becoming stale or rotting in the package. These "manufactured" vegetable **trans** fats are now known to be a major contributing factor in causing heart disease and cancer in America.

The USDA has advised against eating high quality proteins found in animal meats. The smallest part of the "New Food Pyramid," other than fat ingestion is meat and bean consumption. They argue that the cholesterol and saturated fats in these foods cause diseases, especially heart disease. As pointed out in the story of the men of the Lewis and Clark Expedition, this is not the case. These men consumed nearly 20 pounds of animal meat per day and they all lived long lives.

It is not the ingestion of cholesterol or saturated fatty acids per se that create the problem in the human body. If animals consume natural grass and grain feeds, their meat, eggs, and milk are rich in omega-3 fatty acids. If these same animals consume corn silage or soybean meal, (both unnatural foodstuffs for cattle) their meat and dairy products become rich in omega-6 fatty acids. When we eat the animals rich in omega-6 fatty acids, this produces an imbalance of inflammatory and anti-inflammatory factors (prostaglandins, cytokines, leukotrienes, tumor necrosis factor, etc.) in our bodies that cause many deleterious effects to our health. In addition, the effect of chronic ingestion of "manufactured" **trans** fats along with the excess omega-6 fatty acids leads to heart disease, many cancers and chronic inflammatory diseases. I also make this point in my previous book. Greenland Eskimos, Masai and Samburu Indians of Africa all consume diets laden with protein, saturated fats and cholesterol. They have far fewer medical problems than are seen in America and other countries that have adopted the westernized diet (low fat, high carbohydrate, trans fat rich foods). Their diets are also rich in omega-3 fatty acids, contain no manufactured trans fats, and a limited quantity of omega-6 fatty acids.

The present recommendation of the USDA is to eat two fruit, five vegetable and six grain/cereal servings per day. Fruits, vegetables, and grain/cereals are major sources of carbohydrates in our diet. Many of these carbohydrate-rich foods provide various "essential" nutrients discussed earlier that are required for healthy living, but some of these "natural" foods and beverages also provide a large amount of excess fructose that is contributing to several of the health problems facing America at the present time. Additionally, many of the "processed" foods consumed by most of us daily are laden with fructose-rich sugars. In subsequent chapters you will learn how this has happened, the impact it has had on our nation's health, and what you can do to prevent the unhealthy predicaments in your body from regular, excess fructose consumption.

Pearls

- Balanced nutrition is the key to good health.
- The human body needs to regularly consume essential nutrients (water, vitamins, minerals, protein, and fat in the form of omega-3 fatty acid and omega-6 fatty acid) to maintain good health.
- Eliminate all trans fats from the diet as they are the major cause of many diseases.
- The human body does not need carbohydrates to maintain health.
- Present USDA guidelines of a high carbohydrate, low fat diet do not provide the best balance of nutrients required for optimum health.
- Excess fructose in any form is detrimental to the health of the human body.

> **"Variety is the spice of life. That gives it all its flavour."** *William Cowper*

Chapter 4

What Are Carbohydrates?

C arbohydrates are a very large and complex group of carbon- and water-based products found in nature. They are also known as "saccharides" or "sugars" and serve many roles in the chemistry of plants and animals. Carbohydrates are divided into four sizes based on their chemical structure. These include monosaccharides, disaccharides, oligosaccharides and polysaccharides.

The simplest saccharides are the monosaccharides (*mono* = one) as they cannot be broken down to a smaller sugar. The mono-saccharides are the major source of fuel for the metabolism of the body. They include glucose (dextrose), fruit sugar called fructose and galactose. These monosaccharides are also known as simple sugars.

MONOSACCHARIDES (Simple Sugars)
Glucose
Fructose
Galactose

When combined with each other in different pairing combinations, they are the recognizable sugars that we consume. Paired saccharides are called disaccharides (*di* = two). These simple sugars can bind to each other in different patterns, and the position of the binding will change the chemical property of the sugar in major ways. When we find glucose attached to a fructose molecule this becomes sucrose or table sugar. Glucose attached to a galactose molecule is known as lactose or milk sugar. And, when two glucose molecules are attached to each other, they are called maltose or malt sugar and cellulobiose (which is a breakdown product of plant cellulose or plant fiber), depending on how they are connected together.

Maltose and cellulobiose are both disaccharides of glucose, but differ in their attachment. Because of these differing attachments to each other, they have major differences in their ability to be processed by our intestines. The way they are attached to each other is called a chemical bond. The chemical bond is broken down by a specific enzyme.

Maltose is broken down into glucose by enzymes in the small intestine, while cellulobiose passes into the colon where bacteria consume it without providing you with any significant nourishment. The human enzyme system does not have the capability to break the chemical bond found in cellulobiose and many other plant fiber materials. Additionally, the intestine cannot absorb a disaccharide. It must first be broken down into a monosaccharide before the lining of the gut will absorb it and carry it to the liver and bloodstream for furthering the nutritional needs of the human body.

Maltose:	glucose==glucose
	(Very digestible by our intestines)
Cellulobiose:	glucose~~glucose
	(Very *difficult* to digest by our intestines)

As stated, when two monosaccharides are bound to each other they form disaccharides. These sugars, other than the cellulose (or plant fiber) byproducts such as cellulobiose, are digested, absorbed and metabolized by the small intestine, liver and other cells in the human body. Monosaccharides and disaccharides provide immediate energy.

THE COMMON DISACCHARIDES
Sucrose (glucose + fructose)
Lactose (glucose + galactose)
Maltose (glucose + glucose)
Cellulobiose (glucose + glucose)

An enzyme deficiency develops in many people over time that leads to lactose (milk sugar) intolerance. Nearly all humans are born with an enzyme called lactase. This enzyme splits lactose into galactose and glucose. These simple sugars are then transported across the intestinal lining and carried into the bloodstream. When we age, many of us produce less and less lactase, and we can no longer digest milk sugar in the same capacity as when we were breast fed as babies. A deficiency of this enzyme allows more lactose to pass through the small intestine undigested. The sugar makes its way into the colon where bacteria digest it. This lactose digestion leads to the production of colonic gases and acids which produce untoward symptoms for us. These may include: bloating, excessive flatulence, nausea, abdominal cramping and pain, and diarrhea.

When a simple sugar molecule binds to others and forms larger sugars they are known as oligosaccharides (*oligo* = few). They contain between three and nine monosaccharide units bound together. Two interesting oligosaccharides consumed in our diet regularly are raffinose and stachyose. Raffinose is a trisaccharide of glucose, fructose and galactose bound together, while stachyose is raffinose bound to another galactose molecule. These oligosaccharides are found in many vegetables such as beans, cabbage, asparagus, brussel sprouts, and others. These sugars are not metabolized by our intestinal enzymes so they make their way into our colon where bacteria ferment them. The result is the formation of carbon dioxide, methane and/or hydrogen (depending on your gut flora). These are the primary sugars that give us flatus (intestinal gas) when we eat our vegetables.

OLIGOSACCHARIDES
Raffinose: glucose=fructose=galactose
Stachyose: glucose=fructose=galactose=galactose

When the simple sugars are combined into larger molecules they are called polysaccharides (poly = many). The primary polysaccharides found in nature are the starches and plant fibers known as cellulose. Both of these groups of compounds are made up of many glucose molecules attached to each other in repeating patterns. The starch molecules are readily digested by our pancreatic and intestinal enzymes into simpler sugars that can then be absorbed to provide energy to cells throughout the body. The plant fibers (cellulose) are not digestible by our digestive enzyme system because of a different chemical bond structure between the glucose molecules (=) versus (~). When we ingest cellulose and other plant saccharides, they pass into the colon and are fermented by colonic bacteria.

POLYSACCHARIDES:
Starch: glucose=glucose=glucose=etc.
Fiber: glucose~glucose~glucose~etc.

Some of the monosaccharides and disaccharides can be found in their natural alcohol forms (Table 1) and are used to sweeten many foods instead of using table sugar (sucrose).

Table 1. Frequently Consumed Sugar Alcohols Compared With Table Sugar

Compound	Calories (kcal/gram)	Sweetness
Sucrose (Table Sugar)	4.0	1.0
Glycerol	4.3	0.6
Hydrogenated Starch Hydrolysate	3.0	0.4-0.9
Sorbitol	2.6	0.6
Xylitol	2.4	1.0
Maltitol	2.1	2.1
Isomalt	2.0	0.5
Lactitol	2.0	0.4
Erythritol	0.213	0.812
Arabitol	0.2	0.7

Sugar alcohols are typically not as sweet as table sugar, contain fewer calories (Table 1), and do not cause dental cavities. This is because the bacteria that causes tooth decay do not digest these sugar alcohols. In turn, the bacteria do not grow when we eat sugar alcohols and our teeth are spared damage. Some of these compounds are typically not absorbed and make their way into the colon where bacteria ferment them causing us to suffer from bloating, flatulence and diarrhea. One exception to this is erythritol. This sugar alcohol is absorbed but then excreted in the urine unchanged and provides almost no caloric energy to the body.

As can be seen from the table above, some sugar alcohols are nearly as sweet as table sugar. Most contain fewer calories per equal weight amounts. Additionally, beware that *sugar free* does not necessarily mean calorie free when you are substituting sugar alcohols for table sugar or high fructose corn syrup. Their sweetness satisfaction among consumers is highly variable, and many individuals complain of intolerances or side effects from sugar alcohols.

One final note concerning carbohydrates: while plants store glucose in the form of starch (potatoes, rice, grains, etc.), we also have the capacity to store our excess glucose that we have consumed in a molecule known as glycogen. Glycogen is primarily stored in muscle and liver tissue awaiting energy demands by our bodies. As we use our muscles, brain, and other organs, glucose is the primary carbohydrate providing the energy.

Glucose is converted into energy molecules. As the glucose is used up by our bodies, the glycogen reserves are broken down into glucose to maintain a steady energy supply.

When we consume dietary, glucose-containing carbohydrates (table sugar, high fructose corn syrup, starches, etc.) the excess glucose is converted into glycogen until the body can hold no more. We have a limited capacity to store glycogen. Once this short-term storehouse of glycogen is full, the rest of the glucose is converted into fat for long-term storage. Think of the glycogen storehouse as a bottle. When the bottle is filled with glucose, the excess glucose runs over the top of the bottle and is deposited in fat cells. The body's metabolism converts the surplus glucose to fat for long-term storage.

Pearls

- Carbohydrates are a diverse group of sugar molecules found in nature.
- Glucose is the primary carbohydrate supplying energy to the human body.

"Who has never tasted what is bitter does not know what is sweet." *German Proverb*

Chapter 5

Why Sugar?

I f you look at your tongue in the mirror of your bathroom, you will find bumpy little organs that allow you to taste things. These bumps are called taste buds. Taste buds are able to distinguish sweet, bitter, salt and sour. They allow us to recognize various foods and beverages, warn us against dangerous chemicals (such as toxins, poisons, etc.), and bring us pleasure when we partake of various substances.

The sense of taste is enhanced by our sense of smell and touch. Think about the last time you smelled meat sizzling on the barbeque, or walked into the kitchen 30 minutes before the turkey was coming out of the oven on Thanksgiving Day. You can almost taste the food because of your sense of smell. Likewise, the texture of food and beverages adds or detracts from its taste. Coconut immediately comes to mind. If you taste shredded coconut, it tastes different than powdered coconut or a whole piece of coconut meat.

When we taste foods we derive pleasure in various degrees based on the taste bud response to the four flavor sensations mentioned above. The one that has the most powerful effect on the brain is sweet. Studies show that little children can be enticed to look at a camera or follow a person with their eyes by adding sweeteners to their drinking water versus just using water alone. This does not happen when enticing the other taste buds of the little ones.

Sweetness brings us to sugar. Sugars are carbohydrates found in nature that provide plants and animals with a rich source of energy for cellular growth, tissue repair, immune protection and reproduction of offspring.

While it is not impossible to survive without sugar unless you have a rare genetic disorder, eating sugar brings us near instant energy when we consume it. Additionally, our bodies have the metabolic machinery to manufacture sugar when the nutritional needs arise to carry out one of the aforementioned activities.

Our blood sugar (also called glucose or dextrose) level is tightly regulated by insulin and glucagon, two hormones produced by the pancreas. If we develop low blood sugar, we do not feel very well. We have low energy levels; complain of feeling cold, clammy, and shaky; and suffer from headaches. If our blood sugar continues to fall, we develop confusion, hallucinations, seizures, coma and death.

Likewise, we can develop elevated blood sugar levels if we have a lack of insulin or if we develop a tissue resistance to insulin. Elevated blood sugar levels lead to diabetes. Chronically elevated blood sugar levels lead to severe consequences that include kidney damage, blindness, nerve damage, heart disease and premature death.

If our body is working correctly, our blood sugar remains in a stable range regulated by these hormones (insulin and glucagon). This control is influenced by the type of sugars we eat in our diet, the amount of sweets consumed at one time, and the metabolic health of our bodies from past damage inflicted by dietary indiscretions, infections or chronic diseases.

We are born with a natural tendency to prefer sweetness over bitter or sour tastes. Whether we actually develop an addiction or dependence to sugar is a point of contention that has appeared in literature for several decades. One thing is clear: most people enjoy consuming sugar and its various substitutes. Additionally, a comprehensive review of this controversy points out that sugar intake is only indirectly related to diabetes, heart disease, obesity or hyperactivity in children. As I point out in my book concerning fat imbalance, the addition of trans fats and the loss of omega-3 fatty acids in the American diet have been major contributors to these ills, but a component of the sugars we consume in our daily diet of sweets is also causing havoc on our health. That component of our sugars is fructose.

Just what is sugar? If we ask the waitress for sugar to sweeten our ice tea or we go to the grocery store and buy a sack of sugar, what are we eating or buying? Sugar, or table sugar as it has been called for many years, is a carbohydrate found in nature.

The technical name for table sugar is sucrose. Sucrose is a compound composed of two other "sugars" called glucose and fructose. When glucose (also called dextrose) is chemically bound to fructose in a one-to-one ratio, sucrose is the result. Sucrose is found abundantly in sugar beets and sugar cane. Many other fruits and vegetables also contain sucrose; only sugar beets and sugar cane contain high enough concentrations of sucrose for extraction, processing and production of crystalline table sugar.

Sucrose must be extracted from sugar cane or sugar beets by soaking the chopped up plants in hot water. As the sugar is leached out of the plant fibers, a brown liquid known as molasses is formed. Spinning the molasses by high speed centrifuges and then dehydrating the liquid produces brown sugar; removing the brown pigment provides us with table sugar. Varying the size of the sugar crystals as they dry, or grinding to various sizes after the crystals are formed by the dehydration process produces sugars such as powdered sugar, baker's special sugar, fruit sugar, etc. All of these sugars are still just sucrose that varies only according to their texture and crystal size. There are no biochemical differences between any of them.

When our Maker put us together at some time in the distant past, we were blessed with an enzyme that splits table sugar into glucose and fructose. This process occurs in the second portion of the small intestine known as the jejunum. Without this enzyme, we could not digest or absorb table sugar. If we all lacked this enzyme, consumption of table sugar would lead to excessive intestinal gas production, bloating, cramping and diarrhea. Luckily, this enzyme carries out its function or else we would not be able to enjoy our favorite ice cream, candies, cookies, cakes, beverages, etc.

What is important to realize about table sugar is that the glucose and the fructose present are found in a ratio of one-to-one. After sucrose is split into its two simple sugars, they are absorbed across the jejunum and transported to the liver where the metabolic factory of the human body is found. Numerous enzyme systems process the glucose and fructose to produce the many functions I mentioned earlier (cell growth, tissue repair, immune protection, reproduction of offspring). The liver knows exactly what to do with glucose and fructose when they enter it in small quantities in this one-to-one ratio. It is only when this ratio is altered by manufactured sugar (more on this later), too much table sugar, or other sources of fructose that the liver cannot handle the sugar properly. So long as the ratio remains one-to-one of glucose to fructose and in small quantities, we can enjoy sugar without significant ill effects on our diet (except perhaps a contribution to dental cavities).

When the American diet consisted of table sugar as the primary carbohydrate used in sweetening our food, obesity was not a major problem. Obesity has become a major problem only over the past couple of decades, while sugar consumption has been present in the United States for a few centuries.

Natural sugars, such as table sugar, honey, maple syrup and pure corn sugar (glucose and its polymers) have no problem being metabolized by the body in small quantities. We have the biochemical machinery to process them in ways that do not damage the body.

While it is important to remember that we do not need to consume any sugar to stay alive (unless you have a very rare genetic disorder), sugar is one of the major sources of caloric consumption in America. What is fascinating is that sugar consumption was relatively flat at 120 pounds of sugar per capita per year from the 1960s to 1982. With the introduction of high fructose corn syrup, total sugar consumption (table sugar plus high fructose corn syrup) increased to about 150 pounds per year by 2000. This consumption recently has declined and leveled off at around 140 pounds per year by 2005. During the past twenty-five years the consumption of table sugar has decreased by nearly fifty percent while consumption of high fructose corn syrup (HFCS) has increased by over 300% (from almost none in 1970 to nearly 45 pounds per person, per year in 2008).

Mass production of HFCS in the 1970s led to a decrease in the price of sweetened products in the marketplace and a substitution of HFCS for sucrose in many foodstuffs. This replacement has caused a significant increase in intake of sweeteners in general, and fructose specifically (both from table sugar and HFCS).

I hope that by now you realize that table sugar or sucrose per se is not the problem in America. Its steady decline in use over a generation and a half should have led to a decrease in medical problems attributed to its consumption. Unfortunately, the opposite is true. Its intake today is far lower yet we have seen an explosion of diseases attributable to sugar. Medical conditions such as obesity, diabetes, elevated cholesterol, elevated triglycerides, heart disease and high blood pressure have not declined. In fact, all of these conditions have reached epidemic proportions during this time period. The rest of this book will focus on the real culprit causing many of these woes now facing us: That is excess consumption of fructose, independent of its origin. It does not matter whether fructose is derived from table sugar, HFCS, fruits, juices or honey. It is the excess consumption of this simple sugar that is causing serious damage to our health.

Our sweet taste buds have gotten a workout over the past two generations. Now it is time to learn the rest of the story concerning fructose so that we can give them a respite.

Pearls

- Sugar brings much pleasure to most people's diet.
- We prefer sweetness over most other flavors from birth.
- Sugars found in nature consumed in small quantities do not damage the human body.
- Fructose consumption has dramatically increased in the Western diet because of the mass production of high fructose corn syrup.

> **"History is a race between education and catastrophe."** *H.G. Wells*

Chapter 6

The History of Sugar Consumption

The desire to consume sweet foodstuffs dates back to antiquity. First on the scene were sugars consumed in the form of fruits and honey. References date honey gathering to several thousand years ago. Fresh fruit could only be consumed for a few days a year while honey would last for a few months before it would deteriorate beyond palatable human consumption. Fruit would quickly spoil as there was no refrigeration, nitrogen warehouse storage units, freezers or canning to preserve the fruit for consumption another day.

Because fruit could not be kept fresh for any length of time, it was learned that fruit juice could be extracted from the fruit, and the juice could be used to make wines; maltose (malt sugar from barley) could be used to make beer. Honey was used for nourishment, medicine and to sweeten foods. All of these uses occurred before the birth of Christ 2000 years ago.

The use of sugars traveled two pathways: one was for the production of alcoholic beverages, the other was to sweeten foods and beverages. The production of alcoholic products required an understanding of fermentation. Fermentation occurs naturally in nature by various microbiological organisms such as yeast and bacteria. Mankind has always been an experimental creature, and as fermentation was perfected, various fermentation products developed among all regions on Earth. Fermentation is the process of converting a carbohydrate such as fruit sugar into carbon dioxide, energy for the organism fermenting the fruit, alcohol or lactic acid, and water. The fermentation of sugars by yeast (there are some bacteria also) will produce alcohol in the form of wine, cider or beer. If bacteria are utilized in the fermentation process of some sugars, they typically convert these sugars into lactic acid. This results in the production of yogurt, sauerkraut, kimchi, salami, and the like.

Fermentation preceded distillation by at least three millennia, but explorers and travelers crossing trade routes spread the understanding and development of many fermented (and then distilled) beverages that have been refined and mass produced over the centuries.

Distillation is the process of purifying a liquid mixture into its separate components by evaporating the liquid with heat, collecting the vapor, cooling the vapor and re-collecting it in another container. The mixture contains liquids that will evaporate at different temperatures depending on their chemical properties. If the mixture is composed of alcohol and water, such as wine, the water can be removed from the alcohol to produce brandy. The fermentation product of potatoes followed by distillation will make vodka.

Fermentation produces a maximum alcohol content of about 15-20% before the alcohol generated by the yeast or bacteria will kill the organism. Routine distillation techniques can generate alcohol concentrations of near 95%.

At the same time sugars were being used to produce alcohol, sugar cane crops began to flourish in Southeast Asia after people in India discovered how to extract crystalline sugar from the cane around 350 AD. As techniques of table sugar extraction and refining improved, demand for sugar grew rapidly. By the beginning of the last millennium sugar consumption spread across Asia into the eastern Mediterranean, and following the Crusades its use gained popularity throughout Europe.

Christopher Columbus brought sugar plants to the New World in 1492. Over the next two centuries the Caribbean and Central and South America became the largest sugar producers in the world. As the demand for and consumption of sugar (Table 1) increased, so did its production.

Table 1. Sugar Consumption in England by Year

Year	Average Consumption/Year
1700	4 pounds
1800	18 pounds
1850	36 pounds
1900	100 pounds
1960	120 pounds
1980	120 pounds
2000	150 pounds (sugar + HFCS)
2005	140 pounds (sugar + HFCS)

HFCS = High Fructose Corn Syrup

The islands of the Caribbean became major producers of sugar cane until soils became nutritionally depleted. Production then spread to the Americas, and finally the Hawaiian Islands. Sugar cane is still grown in many countries around the globe, but the discovery of high quantities of sugar in sugar beets led to mass production of this crop in the past two centuries.

As can be seen, table sugar is a new food source to the Western world diet in spite of its discovery in Southeast Asia nearly 1500 years earlier. Prior to the discovery of America almost no table sugar was consumed by the common man.

For the next two centuries sugar was still a rare commodity of food and drink. It was only after the product could be grown in abundance, techniques developed to efficiently extract and purify and a means of transport to population centers was made, that sugar could be mass consumed by all of us.

As a side note, sugar refining also was improving in the eighteenth century, and a byproduct of the newer refining techniques was the production of molasses. This then was used in the production of rum and served to increase the demand for even more sugar. Because sugar cane production rapidly depletes the soil of its nutrients, alternative sources of sugar were explored.

In the eighteenth century beets were discovered to contain sugar. As refining techniques improved, sugar beet production expanded and now accounts for nearly 30% of the world's production of sugar. Sugar is now produced in over 120 countries and production exceeds 120 million tons of sugar per year. That is 240,000,000,000 pounds of sugar, which is 40 pounds of sugar for every man, woman and child on the planet.

Pearls

- **Sugar consumption has increased over the past two centuries.**
- **Mass production and improved refining techniques led to increased sugar intake.**
- **Sugar fermentation and distillation have advanced the use of sugar in the world's diet.**

> **"All change is not growth; all movement is not forward."** *Francis Bacon*

Chapter 7

Modern "Sugar" Production

W hen I was a kid growing up in the 1950s and 1960s in north Idaho we did not have free access to sugar. We would be treated with candy at Easter, Halloween and Christmas. We would enjoy the occasional cookie after school, homemade pie after Sunday afternoon dinner, and birthday cake. The rest of the year we did not consume much sugar. Our family would consume at least a gallon of fresh, unpasteurized milk per day and would enjoy fresh fruits in season. Today, fruits and their juices are available 365 days a year. Soda pop, sweetened breakfast cereal, flavored coffees, candy and many other sweets are consumed voraciously on a daily basis by the American public.

My family did not drink soda pop until the 1970s, other than the gallon of A&W root beer enjoyed during haying season. The cost of carbonated beverages was rather expensive in that era. Even though we would pay $1.85 for that gallon of liquid sugar, we would chug it right out of the bottle to cut the hay dust from our parched throats. In 2007 dollars (correcting for inflation) we would pay $9.78 for that same gallon of root beer today. Hence, we rarely drank the beverage.

It is amazing to me that a gallon of A&W root beer costs about $2.00-$3.00 for two 2-liter bottles today, depending on the sale of the week. Let me give you another example of the changes in costs of items to help you understand the differences seen in America over the past several decades.

I bought my first new car in 1972. It was a beautiful four door, "top of the line" Datsun 510. The price tag was all of $2,000. A comparable car today would cost around $10,500 according to inflation conversion tables found on numerous Internet web sites. It would be nearly impossible to purchase a comparable auto at that price today. I recently priced vehicles on the web that would be in the same class as my 1972 Datsun— typical pricing ranges around $18,000.

Why is there such a huge disparity between the changes in the cost of soda pop measured against other commodities like an automobile? The reason is the development of a cheaper form of sweetener known as high fructose corn syrup.

What is high fructose corn syrup? This is a manufactured table sugar "look-alike" that tastes much like table sugar, contains approximately the same number of calories as table sugar and it is far less expensive to produce from corn stalk to sweetener than table sugar. It is so much cheaper that the price of soda pop actually has decreased in price over the past 35 years, while nearly all other commodity prices have risen commensurate with inflation, increased technology, etc.

High fructose corn syrup was first developed in a laboratory in 1958, and industrial production commenced in Japan in the late 1960s. By the late 1970s, high fructose corn syrup made its way into processed foods and beverages in the United States. It is produced by first extracting starch (glucose polymer) from corn and then treating the starch with a fungus known as Aspergillus to break down the glucose polymer into simple glucose. This simple glucose is seen in the grocery stores as corn syrup.

HARVEST **CORN**
↑
MILL **CORN**
↑
EXTRACT **CORN** STARCH
(glucose polymer)
↑
TREAT WITH AMYLASE ENZYME
to shorten glucose polymers
↑
TREAT WITH FUNGUS
to make simple glucose (**CORN** SYRUP)
↑
CONVERT GLUCOSE TO
FRUCTOSE-GLUCOSE MIXTURE
with enzyme extracted from microbes
↑
RE-TREAT
to increase fructose concentration
↑
BLEND CONCENTRATED
FRUCTOSE-GLUCOSE MIXTURE
WITH MORE SIMPLE GLUCOSE
to desired sweetness
↑
HIGH FRUCTOSE **CORN** SYRUP

The corn syrup is then exposed to another chemical process whereupon an enzyme extracted from one of a variety of microbial organisms converts part of the glucose to fructose. The enzyme is glucose isomerase. This produces a fructose-glucose mixture that is then re-treated to increase the fructose concentration to about 90%. This fructose-rich solution is then diluted with more simple sugar (glucose) to produce a mixture that has the desired sweetness.

High fructose corn syrup is adjusted to a specified sweetness by adding various amounts of glucose (corn syrup) to the 90:10 fructose-glucose mixture. For example, soda pop is produced today utilizing a 55:45 fructose-glucose blend as this most closely approximates the taste of table sugar. Because of sugar tariffs imposed by the Carter Administration in 1977 the price of sugar dramatically increased. At the same time the Federal Government provided corn farmers with economic subsidies which opened the door for high fructose corn syrup to become an economically viable alternative to cane and beet sugar. As the technology rapidly advanced, the manufacturing process of high fructose corn syrup improved. This led to decreasing prices for commodities sweetened with high fructose corn syrup compared with table sugar. Over the next three decades more processed foods and beverages utilized high fructose corn syrup. The consumption per capita of high fructose corn syrup surpassed sugar in 2005. The per capita consumption that year was 63 pounds of high fructose corn syrup compared with 59 pounds of table sugar.

In the decade following World War II people consumed only about 10 gallons of soda pop per year. The per capita consumption of sugar-sweetened soda pop was about 18-19 gallons per person per year in 1970 when my family bought A&W root beer. At the present time high fructose corn syrup sweetened soda pop consumption approximates 50 gallons per person per year. The reduced cost of production, sugar tariffs, farm subsidies by the federal government and a powerful sweet tooth have led to this significant increase in sweetener consumption by the American public. We will discuss the ramifications of this increased fructose consumption on our health in subsequent chapters, but suffice it to say, the American public began to gain weight following the introduction of high fructose corn syrup into our daily diet of sweets.

The increase in soda pop consumption is a glaring example of how Americans have increased consumption of fructose sweeteners. But, the truth is that we have increased our intake of other sweets (cookies, candies, cakes, etc.) right along with soda pop since high fructose corn syrup (HFCS) became commercially available for bakers (and the processed food industry) at a very inexpensive price.

One thing that is fascinating about fructose-derived sweetener consumption is that in 1970 the average consumption of these sweeteners was 120 pounds per person, and this was nearly all table sugar and a touch of honey with corn syrup (glucose) thrown in. By 2005 the average American consumption of all fructose products (excluding

Per Capita Consumption of Fructose Derived from Sucrose and HFCS	
1900	15 grams/day
1940	24 grams/day
1977	37 grams/day
1994	55 grams/day
2005	90 grams/day

fruit and fruit juice) had risen to about 135 pounds per year. Fructose consumption from table sugar and HFCS in the United States has increased 500% in the twentieth century, and the majority of that escalation has occurred since the production of high fructose corn syrup in the early 1980's. Was that increase of about 15 pounds of sweetener per year the cause of our problems? Or, is there more to the story of the effects of fructose sweeteners on our health? This issue will be explored later in the book.

Pearls

- Modern sugar production has allowed for the rapid increase in consumption of fructose in our diet.
- High fructose corn syrup (HFCS) is produced from corn syrup and is similar in taste to table sugar.
- Mass production of HFCS has led to the decreased cost of sweetening food products.

"Taste cannot be controlled by law."
Thomas Jefferson

Chapter 8

What is Fructose?

One summer when I was a young parent, I was parboiling some peaches in preparation for peeling and canning them. I set some of the peaches on the dining room table in preparation for the boiling. As I walked back into the kitchen, I heard a slurping sound coming from the dining room. Sitting at the dining room table with a peach in each hand and eating as fast as she could was my little daughter. Juice was dripping from her chin and elbows, but she did not want to stop gulping down every last bite. Why do we love fruit so much? It is because of the fructose in the fruit.

Fructose is a simple monosaccharide (the simplest form of sugar found in nature) sugar that gives fruits, berries, honey, and table sugar their sweetness. How sweet is fructose? Well, it is the sweetest sugar found in nature. It is also much sweeter than table sugar (see table 1). If table sugar is the gold

Table 1. Sweetness of Fructose Compared to Other Common Sugars	
Sugar	**Relative Sweetness**
Fructose	173
Table Sugar	100
Honey	97
Corn Syrup	74
Milk Sugar	16

standard for sweetness with an arbitrary sweetness value of 100, you can see that fructose is significantly sweeter than other common sweeteners.

The fructose found in various food sources is not a sugar that is typically found in its free form on the shelf of your local grocery store. You can find processed fructose in the health food markets or in the nutrition section of some supermarkets.

A controversy surrounds an age-old claim that fructose is habit forming. Some scientists maintain that frequent fructose consumption leads to an intense desire for more fructose. Data now reveal that fructose contributes to both direct and indirect effects on the brain to stimulate your appetite and leave you with a sense of ongoing hunger, even if you have just completed eating a meal.

Because the verdict is not without debate in the food industry, my wife and I decided to withdraw from all fructose-containing foods for three weeks. I felt as though I could not satisfy my appetite no matter how large a meal I consumed for about 5 days. By the end of the first week of my fructose fast, I began to feel full with a normal sized meal, and my craving to continue to eat subsided. My wife felt the same for about 8 days.

I then turned to some nurses that I work with regularly. I convinced some of them to try fasting from fructose for a couple weeks to see what their symptomatic reaction might be. One nurse felt very dizzy for the first 24-36 hours but felt no further symptoms. Another nurse felt much like my wife and I. She always felt hungry, even if she had just completed a meal. This lasted a few days before it finally quit nagging her. Another nurse could not stop consuming fructose in spite of several attempts to fast from the sugar.

The reasons for the symptoms appear to not be just a figment of our imaginations. Data now shows that chronic fructose ingestion leads to the body's resistance to a hormone called leptin. Leptin is a hormone that triggers the brain to remind us that we no longer feel hungry when we are eating. Resistance to leptin causes the body to still feel hungry after completing a meal. In turn, this will cause us to continue to eat and consume too many calories. This may not only be the mechanism that leads to the withdrawal sensations that we went through, it may also be the mechanism that most likely has led to significant weight gain. When our brain is resistant to the signaling of leptin we continue to eat even though we have consumed adequate calories to signal the brain that we have eaten enough food. Animal and human studies reveal that diets rich in fructose (compared with low fructose meals) leads to overeating and weight gain. If animals are fed a fructose-rich diet, they will become obese. If they are then converted back to a fructose-free diet, their appetite and previous weight return to normal. The lack of appetite suppression by leptin while consuming a high fructose diet may be part of the mechanism that is responsible for the significant weight gain we are witnessing in this country today.

We also develop other brain-signaling problems from continued excess fructose ingestion as our body progresses deeper into the metabolic syndrome. Elevated blood triglycerides and insulin resistance also block leptin communication with the brain, and these processes (both manifestations of the metabolic syndrome) leave us with a sense that we are hungry. We will continue to overeat in an attempt to stop that sense of hunger.

The source of fructose is irrelevant to the outcome of leptin resistance and weight gain. The fructose can be in the form of table sugar (sucrose), high fructose corn syrup or simple fructose (found in fruits). The result is the same: overeating and obesity.

Fructose is the only sugar known to cause leptin resistance in the brain. The reason for this is not known, but scientists postulate that it is a mechanism that stimulates appetite during the season of abundance of fructose (fruit season). This overeating in the summer months fattens the body so that it can survive the food shortage that occurs during the winter months. Unfortunately, we now consume excessive amounts of fructose (fruit, fruit juice, soda pop, sweets of all kinds) year-round and never have lean months of food shortage that would reverse the weight gain seen in the fruit season.

Pearls

- Fructose is the sweetest sugar found in nature.
- Chronic, excess fructose ingestion leads to brain resistance of appetite suppression. This leads to overeating and weight gain.
- The source of fructose does not alter this resistance.
- The primary hormone responsible for appetite suppression is leptin.
- Fructose causes the brain to be resistant to leptin signaling.

"The eye sees only what the mind is prepared to comprehend." *Alexander Graham Bell*

Chapter 9

Where Is Fructose Found?

F ructose can be consumed in nature only a few weeks per year in its natural state. Strawberries, raspberries, other berries, and fruit ripen all in a matter of several weeks in the summer. Without the ability to refrigerate, freeze, can or preserve fruits and berries, they quickly spoil and are no longer palatable. Through modern inventions of the last century, we now have the methods to preserve fresh fruit for months in nitrogen warehouses, freeze or freeze-dry fruits, and rapidly transport fruit all over the planet with jet plane travel. This has led to the availability to eat any fruit of our choosing 24:7:365. We are now bathed in fruits and berries, their juices and a plethora of processed products containing their juices.

In addition, there is also the issue of processed foods that have sugar or high fructose corn syrup added for flavoring that will boggle the mind once we start to look for its presence. While this chapter will try to give you an idea of the many sources of fructose in our diet today, I certainly may have missed some of your favorite items. My apologies to you ahead of time. Items are organized into groups of related items. There is also a list of the tables at the back of the book for quick reference.

Table 1. Fructose Content of Alcoholic Beverages

BEVERAGE ALCOHOL	Serving Size	Gm Free Fructose	Grams Sucrose	Total Fructose	Total Sugars
Beer, light	12 oz	0	0	0	0.32
Beer, regular	12 oz	0	0	0	0
Distilled (all)	1.5 oz	0	0	0	0
Rice Sake	1 oz	0	0	0	0
Wine, white	5 oz	Tr	0	Tr	1.41
Wine, red	5 oz	Tr	0	Tr	0.91

As can be seen from Table 1, there is very little fructose in alcohol. Sugar is often added to fortified wines, mixed drinks and dessert wines.

Table 2. Fructose Content of Common Berries

BERRY	Serving Size	Gm Free Fructose	Grams Sucrose	Total Fructose
Blackberry	1 cup	3.46	0.1	3.6
Blueberry	1 cup	7.4	0.2	7.5
Boysenberry	1 cup	4.6	0	4.6
Cranberry	1 cup	0.63	0.13	1.3
Raspberry	1 cup	2.89	0.25	3.1
Strawberry	1 cup	3.71	0.71	4.1

Berries are a major source of fructose. While most of us will not consume a full cup of berries in a single sitting, remember that it is the total amount of fructose that is consumed daily that creates problems with our health. If you only ate a cup of blueberries each day with no other source of fructose, you would be providing yourself with many great nutrients, and you would not be consuming too many grams of fructose for the day. Unfortunately, this is typically only a small portion of our daily intake.

Table 3. Fructose Content of Beverages

BEVERAGE FRUIT/SPORT	Serving Size	Gm Free Fructose	Grams Sucrose	Total Fructose	Total Sugars
Apple Juice	8 oz	14.21	3.12	15.77	23.86
Apple/Grape Juice	8 oz	16.15	1.85	17.08	27.30
Apple/Grape/Pear	8 oz	14.72	1.38	15.41	24.88
Cranberry	8 oz	*	*	*	30.61
Cranberry Cocktail	8 oz	12.57	0	12.57	30.03
Cranberry/Low Cal	8 oz	*	*	*	10.88
Cranberry Diet	8 oz	*	*	*	2.98
Cranberry/Apple	8 oz	*	*	*	35.52
Grape Juice	8 oz	18.62	0.1	18.67	35.93
Grapefruit/Sweeten	8 oz	*	*	*	27.57
Grapefruit	8 oz	*	*	*	21.88
Orange/Unsweeten	8 oz	6.05	10.11	11.11	21.81
Orange/Grapefruit	8 oz	*	*	*	25.14
OJ/Straw/Banana	8 oz	*	*	*	22.42
Pineapple	8 oz	9.53	3.83	11.44	24.95
Pineapple/Grapefruit	8 oz	*	*	*	28.81
Pineapple/Orange	8 oz	*	*	*	28.98
Pomegranate Juice	8 oz	15.86	0	15.86	31.51
Prune Juice	8 oz	*	*	*	42.11
Sport/Gatorade	20 oz	11.08	5.61	13.88	31.91
Sport/Powerade	12 oz	11.75	0.73	12.12	22.31
Sport/Propel	12 oz	*	*	*	4.34
Tomato Juice	8 oz	3.74	0.61	4.05	8.65
V8 Juice	8 oz	*	*	*	7.99
V8 Fusion	8 oz	*	*	*	26.01
V8 Splash	8 oz	*	*	*	19.01

* No data available

Most juices and sport drinks provide excessive amounts of fructose and are not tolerated in any quantity in our diet. Even reasonable quantities of these beverages contain so much fructose that we quickly exceed our daily metabolic capacity for this sugar. Our liver can only tolerate 12-18 grams of fructose per day (12-15 for females, 15-18 for males) without creating chaos in the chemistry of our metabolism.

Table 4. Fructose Content of Bread

BREAD	Serving Size	Gm Free Fructose	Grams Sucrose	Total Fructose	Total Sugars
French	1 slice	0	0	0	1.64
Italian	1 slice	0	0	0	0
Multi-Grain	1 slice	0.64	0	0.64	1.66
Oatmeal	1 slice	*	*	*	2.21
Pita	1 small	*	*	*	0.36
Pumpernickel	1 slice	*	*	*	0.14
Raisin	1 slice	*	*	*	1.88
Rye	1 slice	*	*	*	1.23
Sourdough	1 slice	0	0	0	1.64
Wheat	1 slice	*	*	*	1.44
White	1 slice	0.46	0	0.46	1.08

No data available

Breads are basically a very safe part of the Western diet. While they provide us with carbohydrates, they do not add much fructose to our daily intake. The exceptions to this are white, multigrain and raisin breads. This is because sugars have been added to sweeten them. Be sure and check the ingredient section of the food label to see what sugars have been added to the bread for this purpose.

Table 5. Fructose Content of Breakfast Cereals

BREAKFAST CEREAL	Serving Size	Gm Free Fructose	Grams Sucrose	Total Fructose	Total Sugars
All Bran	1 cup	0.11	4.09	2.16	4.91
Apple Jacks	1 cup	0.22	13.18	6.81	13.72
Cheerios	1 cup	0	1.13	0.56	1.13
Cinnamon Crunch	3/4 cup	2.25	7.58	6.04	10.28
Corn Flakes	1 cup	0.38	1.14	0.95	2.94
Corn Grits	1 cup	0	0.31	0.16	0.31
Cornmeal	1 cup	0.29	1.16	0.87	2.61
Cream of Rice	1 cup	0	0	0	0
Cream of Wheat	1 cup	0	0.07	0.04	0.11
Froot Loops	1 cup	*	*	*	12.47
Frosted Flakes	3/4 cup	0.37	10.69	5.72	11.62
Frosted Mini Wheats	1 cup	*	*	*	10.71
Granola	1 cup	*	*	*	24.01
Grape Nuts	1/2 cup	0.49	0	0.49	7.29
Honey Nut Cheerios	3/4 cup	*	*	*	9.01
Lucky Charms	1 cup	0.15	11.57	5.94	14.01
Mueslix	2/3 cup	*	*	*	17.11
Oatmeal Crisp, Raisin	1 cup	*	*	*	20.31
Oatmeal, Hot	1 cup	0	0.68	0.34	1.11
Puffed Wheat	3/4 cup	0	0	0	0
Raisin Bran	1 cup	*	*	*	18.31
Rice Chex	1 cup	0	0	0	2.01
Rice Krispies	1 cup	0.15	2.33	1.32	2.65
Special K	1 cup	*	*	*	4.01
Total	3/4 cup	*	*	*	5.01
Trix	1 cup	*	*	*	12.01
Wheat Chex	3/4 cup	*	*	*	4.71
Wheaties	3/4 cup	*	*	*	3.61

* No data available

Cereals are another rich source of fructose. It is also important to realize a serving size is much smaller than typically consumed by most children in America. You could easily double that amount for a typical bowl of cereal, especially for teenagers.

Table 6. Fructose Content of Cheese

CHEESE	Serving Size	Gm Free Fructose	Grams Sucrose	Total Fructose	Total Sugars
American	1 slice	*	*	*	0.12
Blue	1 oz	*	*	*	0.14
Brie	1 oz	*	*	*	0.13
Cheddar	1 slice	0	0.07	0.04	0.15
Colby	1 slice	*	*	*	0.15
Cottage, 2%	1 cup	0	0	0	8.29
Cottage	1 cup	0	0	0	5.61
Cream	1 tbsp	0	0	0	0.47
Feta	1 oz	*	*	*	1.16
Fontina	1 slice	*	*	*	0.43
Goat	1 oz	*	*	*	0.25
Gouda	1 oz	*	*	*	0.63
Gruyere	1 slice	*	*	*	0.11
Limberger	1 oz	*	*	*	0.14
Monterey	1 slice	*	*	*	0.14
Mozzarella	1 oz	0.04	0.01	0.05	0.29
Muenster	1 slice	*	*	*	0.31
Parmesan	1 oz	0.04	0.04	0.05	0.26
Provolone	1 slice	*	*	*	0.16
Ricotta	1/2 cup	*	*	*	0.33
Romano	1 oz	*	*	*	0.21
Roquefort	1 oz	*	*	*	
Swiss	1 slice	0	0.04	0.02	0.37

* No data available

Cheeses are fructose free for the most part. You will have noticed by now that there are many data points missing (no data). All of the data was extracted from the Food and Drug Administration web site (see bibliography), and they do not provide specific sugar contents for many foods and beverages.

Table 7. Fructose Content of Condiments

CONDIMENTS	Serving Size	Gm Free Fructose	Grams Sucrose	Total Fructose	Total Sugars
Almond Butter	2 tbsp	0	0	0	2.01
Barbeque Sauce	1 tbsp	4.32	0.04	4.34	9.62
Butter	1 tsp	0	0	0	0
Horseradish	1 tsp	0	0	0	0
Jams, Varieties	1 tbsp	*	*	~4.01	9.75
Jellies, Varietes	1 tbsp	*	*	~5.01	10.82
Ketchup	1 tbsp	1.39	0	1.39	3.41
Mayonnaise	1 tbsp	0	0	0	0
Mustard	1 tsp	0.01	0.01	0.01	0.01
Mustard, Dijon	1 tsp	*	*	*	2.01
Mustard, Honey	1 oz	*	*	*	5.01
Olives, All	1 oz	0	0	0	0
Peanut Butter	2 tbsp	0	0	0	1.01
PB/Sugar Add	2 tbsp	0	1.34	0.67	2.71
Pickle, Dill	1 small	0.16	0	0.16	0.49
Pickle, Sweet	1 small	1.32	0	1.32	2.71
Relish/Sweet	1 tbsp	*	*	*	4.38
Soy Sauce	1 tsp	0	0	0	0
Worcestershire	1 tbsp	*	*	*	1.71

* No data available

Jams, jellies, barbeque sauces, ketchup, sweet pickles and sweet relish are a rich source of fructose.

Table 8. Fructose Content of Entrees

ENTREES	Serving Size	Gm Free Fructose	Grams Sucrose	Total Fructose
Bacon	3 oz	0	0	0
Beef, All Cuts	4 oz	0	0	0
Chicken, All Cuts	4 oz	0	0	0
Cornish Hen	4 oz	0	0	0
Crabs, All Types	3 oz	0	0	0
Eggs, All Types	1 egg	0	0	0
Fish, Freshwater	3 oz	0	0	0
Fish, Saltwater	3 oz	0	0	0
Goose	4 oz	0	0	0
Lobster, All Types	3 oz	0	0	0
Pork, All Cuts	4 oz	0	0	0
Salami, All Types	1 oz	0	0	0
Sausage, Beef	3 oz	0	0	0
Sausage, Pork	3 oz	0	0	0
Shrimp, All Types	3 oz	0	0	0
Turkey	4 oz	0	0	0
Wild Game Meat	4 oz	0	0	0

Eggs and meats of all types (other than sweeten meats such as jerky, Teriyaki, etc.) do not contain fructose or any other carbohydrate. Check the food label for the sugar content of sweetened meats. These foods are healthy for consumption so long as the animal has been fed a diet rich in omega-3 fatty acids (grasses, flax meal, algae from the sea, etc.). These entrees are the major source of protein for most Americans unless you are a vegan. The condiments and other sources of carbohydrates that accompany the entrée are typically where many grams of fructose will be added to a meal.

Table 9. Fructose Content of Fruit

FRUIT	Serving Size	Gm Free Fructose	Grams Sucrose	Total Fructose
Apple	1 medium	10.7	3.8	12.6
Apricot	1 fruit	0.3	2.1	1.4
Avocado	1 cup	0.18	0.14	0.3
Banana	1 large	6.6	3.25	8.2
Cantaloupe	1/2 melon	5.2	12	11.2
Cherries, Sweet	1 cup	7.4	0.2	7.5
Cherries, Sour	1 cup	5.4	1.2	6.1
Coconut, meat	1 cup	0.2	4.5	2.5
Dates, Soft-Medjool	1 date	7.67	0.13	7.7
Dates, Deglet Noor	1 date	1.37	1.67	2.2
Grapefruit/Any	1/2 melon	2.17	4.32	4.3
Grapes, green/red	10 grapes	3.98	0.74	4.3
Guava	1 fruit	0.38	0.38	0.6
Kiwi Fruit	1 medium	3.3	0.11	3.4
Lemon	1 fruit	0.8	0.6	1.1
Lime	1 fruit	0.12	0	0.1
Mango	1 fruit	2.9	9.9	7.9
Nectarine	1 medium	1.95	6.92	4.39
Orange, Navel	1 fruit	3.71	7.06	7.24
Papaya	100 grams	2.7	1.8	3.6
Peach	1 medium	2.29	7.14	6.9
Pear	1 medium	11.09	1.38	11.8
Pineapple	1 cup	3.49	9.88	8.4
Plum	1 medium	2.03	1.04	2.5
Pomegranate	1 medium	13.16	1.12	13.7
Purple Passion Fruit	1 fruit	0.56	0.59	0.8
Rhubarb	1 cup	0.18	0.16	0.3
Starfruit	1 medium	3.2	0.8	3.6
Tangerine	1 medium	2.11	5.32	4.8
Watermelon	1 wedge	9.61	3.46	11.5

Fruits, like fruit juices, are another major source of fructose. While fruit is not bad for our health in moderation, the body can only metabolize about 12-18 grams of fructose per day (12-15 per female, 15-18 per male) without turning on chemical processes that lead to many medical problems. As can be seen by the above table, a medium sized apple has enough fructose to meet the upper limit of daily fruit sugar without adding any further sugar. The new guidelines put out to the American public by the U. S. Department of Agriculture "Food Pyramid" suggests that we consume two to three times that quantity of fruit per day. This was reiterated in the recently released President's Task Force on Childhood Obesity recommendations. As you can see from the fruit table, you will quickly surpass your daily limit of fructose if you follow either of these guidelines. What's more, this will lead directly to obesity and a deranged metabolism.

Limes, rhubarb and lemons are low in fructose. Because of this, many dishes or beverages add table sugar or high fructose corn syrup in order to make them more palatable. This is defeating if you are trying to keep your fructose intake to a minimum.

Avocado, while a fruit, is consumed as a vegetable. We do not sweeten this fruit before it is consumed. This becomes a valuable fruit in your diet for a source of many essential vitamins and minerals without consuming excess fructose.

Watermelon, apples, pears and cantaloupe contain nearly a complete daily dose of fructose in a single serving and are difficult to include in a diet that maintains a low quantity of fructose. As can be discerned from the fruit table, fruit is nothing more than nature's candy. Most fruits should be consumed more as a treat than a daily staple to your diet if you want to prevent the metabolic consequences of excess fructose intake.

Table 10. Fructose Content of Herbs

HERBS	Serving Size	Gm Free Fructose	Grams Sucrose	Total Fructose
Basil	1/4 cup	0	0	0
Cilantro	1/4 cup	0	0	0
Dill	1 tbsp	0	0	0
Fennel	1 tbsp	*	*	*
Marjoram	1 tbsp	*	*	0.01
Oregano	1 tsp	0.02	0.02	0.03
Parsley	1 tbsp	*	*	0.02
Rosemary	1 tbsp	0	0	0
Sage	1 tbsp	0	0	0
Tarragon	1 tsp	0.04	0.04	0.06
Thyme	1 tsp	0	0	0
No data available				

Herbs add a great deal of flavor to foods without adding any significant fructose to your diet.

Table 11. Fructose Content of Mushrooms

MUSHROOM	Serving Size	Gm Free Fructose	Grams Sucrose	Total Fructose	Total Sugars
Chanterelle	1 cup	0	0	0	0
Morel	1 cup	0	0	0	0
Portabella	1 cup	0.42	0	0.42	2.15
Shiitake	1 cup	0	0	0	0
White	1 cup	0.12	0	0.12	1.39

When mushrooms are consumed as a flavorful addition to a steak or as a component to a sauce or gravy, very little fructose is added.

Table 12. Fructose Content of Non-Alcoholic Beverages

BEVERAGES NON-ALCOHOL	Serving Size	Gm Free Fructose	Grams Sucrose	Total Fructose
Coffee	1 cup	0	0	0
Cola, No Caffeine	12 oz	22.45	0	22.45
Cola, Caffeine	12 oz	22.45	0	22.45
Lemonade	1 cup	10.5	11.76	16.38
Milk, Nonfat	1 cup	0	0	0
Milk, 1%	1 cup	0	0	0
Milk, 2%	1 cup	0	0	0
Milk, Whole	1 cup	0	0	0
Sprite, No Caffeine	12 oz	19.15	2.41	20.35
Sprite, Caffeine	12 oz	21.66	0	21.66
Tea, Black	1 cup	0	0	0
Tea, Green	1 cup	0	0	0
Tea, White	1 cup	0	0	0

Non-alcoholic beverages do not provide any fructose unless they are sweetened by sugar or high fructose corn syrup. If you enjoy a morning cup of coffee or tea, the only fructose you will consume is the sweetener you add for flavor. That grande latte, cappuccino, or mocha on the way to work or while strolling around the mall, likewise does not contain fructose unless you have had it doctored with sweeteners contained in the syrups or sugar used to flavor the coffee drink.

Soda pop contains a very large quantity of fructose. With the bad press that is presently surrounding high fructose corn syrup (HFCS), some beverage companies have taken advantage of this to promote HFCS-free drinks. The problem with this is that these sugar sweetened sodas still contain about 20 grams of fructose per twelve ounce container. This still far exceeds the daily amount tolerated by the liver. The only way that soda pop can be included in your diet would be to consume sugar-free forms.

Table 13. Fructose Content of Nuts

NUTS	Serving Size	Gm Free Fructose	Grams Sucrose	Total Fructose
Almonds	1/4 cup	0.03	1.29	0.67
Brazil	1/4 cup	0	0.78	0.39
Cashews	1/4 cup	0.08	1.21	0.68
Filberts	1/4 cup	0.02	1.35	0.69
Macadamia	1/4 cup	0.02	1.13	0.57
Pecans	1/4 cup	0.01	1.11	0.56
Pine Nuts	1/4 cup	0.02	0.98	0.51
Pistachios	1/4 cup	0.04	2.06	1.07
Walnut,Black	1/4 cup	0.01	0.28	0.18
Walnut,English	1/4 cup	0.03	0.69	0.37

Table 13 points out that nuts contain a small amount of fructose per serving. Nuts contain numerous beneficial components to health while they quickly suppress our appetite. They also contain omega-3 fatty acids which are beneficial to the heart— several studies have demonstrated this fact. Data now suggests that regular consumption of nuts typically adds two to three years to your life.

These tasty morsels also contain a rich source of protein, fiber, essential vitamins, minerals and antioxidants. They are an excellent snack food which helps keep us away from excess fructose intake. Peanuts are not included in the list as they are not technically a nut, but they do not contain fructose.

Nuts are consumed by themselves or as additions to main dishes and desserts.

Table 14. Fructose Content of Spices

SPICES	Serving Size	Gm Free Fructose	Grams Sucrose	Total Fructose
Allspice	1 tsp	*	*	*
Anise	1 tsp	*	*	*
Caraway	1 tsp	*	*	*
Celery	1 tsp	*	*	*
Chili Powder	1 tsp	0.11	0.02	0.13
Cinnamon	1 tsp	0.03	0	0.03
Cloves	1 tsp	0.02	0	0.02
Cumin	1 tsp	*	*	*
Curry	1 tsp	0.02	0.01	0.03
Garlic	1 tsp	0.01	0.06	0.04
Mustard	1 tsp	0	0.07	0.04
Onion	1 tsp	0.04	0.09	0.09
Paprika	1 tsp	0.14	0.02	0.15
Pepper,Black	1 tsp	*	*	*
Pepper,Red	1 tsp	*	*	*
Poppy Seed	1 tsp	0.01	0.07	0.05
Poultry Seas.	1 tsp	*	*	*
Turmeric	1 tsp	0.01	0.05	0.04

* No data available

Spices, like herbs, are wonderful additions to the flavoring of prepared foods and beverages. They contain almost no fructose. Most spices add medicinal benefits as well, but that is far beyond the scope of this book. It is safe to say that while some of the spices listed in the above table have no data available on fructose content, they also contain no significant amount of this sugar.

Table 15. Fructose Content of Starches

STARCHES	Serving Size	Gm Free Fructose	Grams Sucrose	Total Fructose	Total Sugars
Couscous	1 cup	0	0	0	0.16
Noodles, egg	1 cup	0	0.06	0.03	0.64
Macaroni	1 cup	0.03	0.1	0.08	0.64
Potato, hashed	1 cup	0.81	0.51	1.06	2.32
Potato, russet	1 cup	0.17	0.1	0.22	0.47
Potato, white	1 cup	0.72	0.6	0.75	2.45
Rice, brown	1 cup	0	0.68	0.34	0.68
Rice, Chinese	1 cup	0	0.46	0.23	0.59
Rice, white	1 cup	0.03	0.13	0.09	0.17
Spaghetti	1 cup	0.04	0.13	0.11	0.78
Sweet potato	1 cup	0.66	2.98	2.15	11.09
Wild rice	1 cup	0.33	0.54	0.61	1.21
Yam	1 cup	0.01	0.01	0.02	0.75

Table 15 is very important for you to study and apply to your food consumption. As can be seen, most starch-rich foods contain very little fructose. As I pointed out earlier in this book, starches are glucose molecules attached to each other. Noodles, rice and potatoes contain very limited amounts of fructose.

Sweet potatoes contain quite a bit of fructose per serving, but can be incorporated into your diet if you watch the rest of your total daily fructose intake. Yams would be a better alternative.

An important point to remember is that if you are a fan of french fries, you will consume 1.4 grams of fructose per tablespoon of ketchup while eating only 0.22 grams of fructose for the entire serving of your russet fries.

Table 16. Fructose Content of Sweeteners

SWEETENERS	Serving Size	Gm Free Fructose	Grams Sucrose	Total Fructose
Corn Syrup	1 tsp	0	0	0
Honey	1 tbsp	8.59	0.19	8.69
Molasses	1 tbsp	2.56	5.88	5.59
Sugar, Brown	1 tsp	0	4.2	2.1
Sugar, Powdered	1 tsp	0	4.2	2.1
Sugar, Table	1 tsp	0	4.2	2.1

When I was a kid one of my favorite treats at Halloween time was popcorn balls. My mom would make these delicious treats every year. As I learned many years later, popcorn balls were made with corn syrup. This sweetener contains no fructose— its only ingredients are glucose, salt and vanilla flavoring. While corn syrup is not as sweet as table sugar or high fructose corn syrup, it does not add to our daily intake of fructose.

Honey and molasses are rich sources of fructose. Because of this, they should be removed from daily consumption in a low fructose diet unless ingested in very small quantities.

Sugar preparations contain the same amount of fructose independent of the form in which they are prepared. They all contain 50% fructose and 50% glucose by weight. As can be seen from the table, sugar is the best bet for sweetening pastries or beverages other than corn syrup when trying to keep your fructose intake to a minimum. A teaspoonful of table sugar contains 1.2 grams of fructose. One teaspoonful of high fructose corn syrup contains 1.65 grams of fructose.

The next four tables contain a large number of vegetables. I have organized them into leafy, root, sprouting and vine varieties in order to break them up into smaller lists.

While vegetables contain fructose, only select ones such as sugar beets, green peas and sweet corn contain enough to pay attention to in planning your daily fructose intake. Even then, most of us do not consume a full cup of a vegetable when served with a meal. Because of this, vegetables are an excellent source of minerals and vitamins while providing a wide variation in our diet.

Table 17. Fructose Content of Leafy Vegetables

VEGETABLE LEAFY	Serving Size	Gm Free Fructose	Grams Sucrose	Total Fructose	Total Sugars
Cabbage,Chinese	1 cup	*	*	*	0.83
Cabbage, raw	1 cup	1.01	0.06	1.04	2.24
Cabbage, red	1 cup	1.04	0.42	1.25	2.68
Cabbage, savoy	1 cup	*	*	*	1.59
Collards	1 cup	*	*	*	0.17
Kale	1 cup	*	*	*	*
Lettuce, bibb	1 cup	0.28	0	0.28	0.52
Lettuce, romaine	1 cup	0.68	0	0.68	1.01
Lettuce, green	1 cup	0.15	0	0.15	0.28
Lettuce, iceberg	1 cup	0.89	0.04	0.93	1.75
Lettuce, red	1 cup	0.24	0	0.24	0.41
Rhubarb	1 cup	*	*	*	1.34
Spinach	1 cup	0.04	0.02	0.05	0.13

* *No data available*

Table 18. Fructose Content of Root Vegetables

VEGETABLE ROOT	Serving Size	Gm Free Fructose	Grams Sucrose	Total Fructose	Total Sugars
Beets, sugar	1 cup	0.79	25	13.35	28.26
Carrots,raw	1 medium	0.34	2.19	1.44	2.89
Ginger root	1 tsp	*	*	*	0.03
Kohlrabi	1 cup	*	*	*	3.51
Onion,raw	1 slice	0.49	0.38	0.66	1.61
Onion,scallion	1 cup	*	*	*	2.33
Onion,sweet	1 cup	2.02	0.72	2.38	5.02
Onion,green	1 cup	1.91	0.14	1.98	3.51
Onion,yellow	1 cup	1.29	0.71	1.35	
Parsnips	1 cup	*	*	*	6.38
Radishes	1/2 cup	0.41	0.06	0.44	1.08
Rutabagas	1 cup	*	*	*	7.84
Turnips	1/2 cup	*	*	*	2.47

* No data available

Table 19. Fructose Content of Sprouting Vegetables

VEGETABLE SPROUTING	Serving Size	Gm Free Fructose	Grams Sucrose	Total Fructose	Total Sugars
Artichoke	1 medium	0.02	0.88	0.46	1.19
Asparagus	1 cup	0.71	0.07	0.75	1.17
Broccoli	1/2 cup	0.58	0.06	0.61	1.08
Brussel sprouts	1/2 cup	*	*	*	1.36
Cauliflower	1 cup	1.04	0	1.04	2.04
Celery	1 cup	0.52	0.11	0.58	1.85
Corn, sweet	1 medium	1.98	0.91	2.43	6.39
Garlic	1 clove	*	*	*	0.03

* No data available

Table 20. Fructose Content of Vine Vegetables

VEGETABLE VINE	Serving Size	Gm Free Fructose	Grams Sucrose	Total Fructose	Total Sugars
Bean,Green	1 cup	0.52	0.25	0.64	1.71
Bean,Lima	1/2 cup	*	*	*	1.15
Bean,Navy	1 cup	0	0.44	0.22	*
Bean,Pinto	1 cup	0	3.82	1.91	*
Bean,Red	1 cup	0	4.74	2.37	*
Bean,White	1 cup	*	*	*	*
Eggplant	1 cup	*	*	*	3.17
Pea,Green	1 cup	0.57	7.24	4.19	8.22
Pepper,Chili	1 cup	*	*	*	2.31
Pepper,Jalepeno	1 cup	*	*	*	3.11
Pepper,Green	1 cup	1.67	0.13	1.73	2.86
Pepper,Red	1 cup	3.37	0	3.37	6.26
Pumpkin,Raw	1 cup	*	*	*	1.58
Pumpkin,Canned	1 cup	*	*	*	8.09
Squash,Summer	1 cup	1.07	0.03	1.09	2.49
Squash,Winter	1 cup	*	*	*	4.04
Squash,Zucchini	1 cup	*	*	*	3.82
Tomato (fruit)	1 slice	0.27	0	0.27	0.53

* No data available

Vegetables (other than beets) only become a significant source of fructose when we combine condiments such a honey mustard dressing with a salad or sugar sauce to a cabbage slaw. The other way is when our diet combines several vegetables, beans and fruits together in salads, smoothies and salsas.

Most of us have never paid much attention to the fructose content of the foods we consume on a daily basis. While government agencies, the media and bloggers focus on their dietary pet peeves, very little attention has been paid to the sources of fructose in our diet. Various groups point the finger at saturated fat, cholesterol, high fructose corn syrup, salt, trans fats or excess calories. Some of these have their problems in our diet, but the one substance that dramatically and consistently deranges the metabolism of the human body is fructose. When consumed in excess of 12-18 grams per day (12-15 per female, 15-18 per male) the body's metabolism changes (see next two chapters). If we are unaware of the fructose content in our food, we can make little progress to improve our health in any meaningful way.

While it is important to eliminate trans fats from our diet in order to reduce our risk of cancer and heart disease, it is also important to consume omega-3 fatty acids and omega-6 fatty acids in a two-to-one ratio to keep our immune system strong, and balance the inflammatory and anti-inflammatory systems of the body (see my previous book for a detailed explanation). Likewise, excess calorie intake and salt intake are not healthy. But, the biggest plague to destruction of our health is excess fructose consumed on a daily basis. These food tables will help you see where you can make changes in your diet to reduce daily fructose intake to a moderate level.

Pearls

- Fructose is found in many food products in our diet.
- Most of us are unaware of how much fructose we consume daily.
- Very few foods contain no fructose.
- Fruits, juices and sugar and high fructose corn syrup-sweetened foods and beverages contain the most significant amounts of fructose in our diet.

"Nothing in life is to be feared. It is to be only understood." *Marie Curie*

Chapter 10

Understanding the Metabolic Syndrome

When I was a kid growing up in small town America, none of my buddies had any fat on their bodies (to speak of). Sure, we had big and little guys, but nobody was obese. To validate my memory I only have to look at my high school yearbooks— the evidence is documented in the photographs of my youth. Today, the scene in our culture is dramatically different. Why has the American public at large gained so much weight?

When we set out to discover the answer to this question we first need to look to the medical profession and medical science in general. Medical investigators across America have come to realize that many health problems are associated with obesity. And, many overweight or obese individuals have a cluster of symptoms and medical conditions associated with excess weight. It is becoming much clearer that medical problems and symptoms and obesity go hand-in-hand; but obesity per se does not cause the symptoms and problems. They are caused by a common driving force, and we will discuss this further in the next chapter.

The purpose of this chapter is to help you understand the cluster of symptoms and medical problems as a specific entity before we explore the cause. First, it is important to understand that when health care professionals combine a group of symptoms or medical problems together to arrive at a diagnosis, the cluster of symptoms can be given a specific name like asthma, influenza, myocardial infarction (heart attack) or hemochromatosis (a genetically inherited excess iron storage disease).

Sometimes, the cluster of symptoms and medical problems does not have a specific diagnostic name so its sum total of findings is called a syndrome. This is the case for a syndrome first described in 1947, but still not completely defined in spite of intense scientific investigation over the past 30 years. Part of the reason that it has taken so long to figure out how to define this particular syndrome is that the various components of the syndrome may have multiple and independent causes which have nothing to do with this specific syndrome. For example, there may be several causes of high blood pressure. Yet, high blood pressure is now recognized as a component of this syndrome. Likewise, there are several causes of elevated blood levels of triglycerides (a type of fat). The high serum triglyceride found in most individuals is part of this syndrome. The challenge is to see how the components of the syndrome are linked together from a common origin rather than being identified as a specific disease present in an individual.

A person can suffer from an inherited form of elevated serum triglycerides, have obesity from chronic, excess fat intake, and be a victim of high blood pressure because of a narrowing of a blood vessel leading to the kidney, yet that individual may not be suffering from a syndrome that contains all three components of the syndrome. These abnormalities found in this individual are unrelated to each other, and so the person would not be considered to be suffering from the syndrome. Rather, he or she would have three separate and independent diseases with specific causes for each diagnosis.

It is becoming clear that there is a cluster of conditions that are interrelated and are strongly associated with the obesity problem that is affecting so many Americans today. This syndrome that is related to the rapidly rising obesity crisis in America is now called the *metabolic syndrome*, but it has had various names ascribed to it in the medical literature that include:

Diabesity
Syndrome X
Insulin Resistance Syndrome
Dysmetabolic Syndrome
Metabolic Syndrome X
Reaven's Syndrome
Visceral Obesity Syndrome

Regardless of the variety of synonyms, what is the *metabolic syndrome*? This syndrome by the United States National Cholesterol Education Program Adult Treatment Panel III (2001) is defined as a clustering of **at least three of the five following symptoms and/or medical problems** that increase your risk of developing insulin-resistant diabetes, heart disease and stroke.

The five components of the *metabolic syndrome* include:

(1) **Increased abdominal girth**
Greater than 40 inch waistline for men
Greater than 35 inch waistline for women
(2) **High blood pressure**
Systolic Pressure greater than 130 mm Hg (top number of your blood pressure)

Diastolic Pressure greater than 85 mm Hg (bottom number of blood pressure)

(3) **Elevated fasting blood sugar (Type II Diabetes, Insulin Resistance, Impaired Glucose Intolerance)**
(Fasting blood glucose greater than 110 mg/dl)

(4) **Elevated serum triglyceride level**
(Greater than 150 gm/dl)

(5) **Low level of HDL cholesterol**
(Good cholesterol)
Less than 40 mg/dl for men
Less than 50 mg/dl for women

Typical of syndromes, numerous international organizations define the metabolic syndrome, each having a variation on this theme for a number of reasons. I will not outline all of the minor differences in the definitions for each group, but they do not deviate from the central concept of abdominal obesity, impaired glucose tolerance, high blood pressure, elevated triglycerides and reduced HDL (good) cholesterol.

Syndromes remain syndromes until a cause can be determined, at which point the cluster of symptoms and medical problems can be given a specified name. As science and technology advance the knowledge of medicine, the cause of the syndrome becomes better understood. The same is true for the *metabolic syndrome.*

While the metabolic syndrome was rare until the past couple decades, it now affects over a third of the adult population and a rapidly increasing percentage of our youth. As the metabolic syndrome reaches epidemic proportions in America its effects are impacting our nation's health in many ways. We will explore this further in another chapter.

Controversy surrounds the metabolic syndrome by some organizations and scientists. An individual can have significant peripheral obesity without abdominal obesity and not be plagued by the metabolic syndrome. Likewise, another can be lean without central obesity but still suffer from the syndrome.

The next chapter will explore the present state of our understanding of this syndrome as it relates to sugar inges- tion and the obesity epidemic sweeping across our nation.

Pearls

- The metabolic syndrome is a group or cluster of medical conditions now affecting one third of the adult population.

  ○ Increased Abdominal Girth
  ○ High Blood Pressure
  ○ Elevated Fasting Blood Sugar (Type II Diabetes)
  ○ Elevated Serum Triglycerides
  ○ Low Level of HDL Cholesterol

- This syndrome is increasing in epidemic proportion and is now affecting the youth of America.

**"I hear and I forget. I see and I remember.
I do and I understand."** *Confucius*

Chapter 11

Fructose and the
Metabolic Syndrome

B enjamin Franklin is credited with the saying, "An apple a day keeps the doctor away" in his writings found in *Poor Richard's Almanack* of the eighteenth century. While this proverb is at least 250 years old, insights into the metabolic effects of the sugar found in an apple are only now being unraveled. You see, apples are loaded with fructose. The focus of this chapter is to provide an understanding of what happens to that fructose when we eat that apple (or many apple equivalents) every day.

If you eat a medium-sized apple each day, you are consuming about 12-13 grams of fructose. A large apple may contain over 20 grams of this fruit sugar. This fructose is converted to glucose by the liver. The liver can then send the glucose to the body's organs where it is converted to ATP (the energy that runs the body, much like gasoline runs a car). Alternatively, if the body has excess glucose around, the excess is stored as glycogen until the body demands more energy.

The medical literature reveals that this small quantity of fructose does not alter the normal biology of the human body. A minor amount of fructose on a daily basis seems to be safe for human consumption so long as we are not consuming excess calories in general. Additionally, if we overindulge and eat five apples (or their equivalent) in a single sitting, we get a bellyache, nausea, cramping, bloating, and diarrhea. The reason for this is that the excess fructose ingested in a large, single ingestion leads to fructose malabsorption. The excess fructose cannot be absorbed fast enough and makes its way into our colon, where bacteria eat the sugar and gastrointestinal symptoms ensue. A single overindulgent fructose meal does not cause any changes in the metabolism of our bodies.

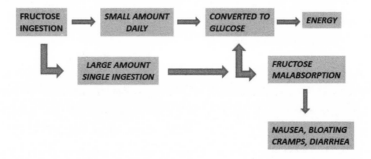

What happens if you begin to consume large amounts of fructose daily? For example: a 12 ounce glass of orange juice (32 grams of sugar) and a toasted frosted raspberry popup (19 grams of sugar) for breakfast, a medium-sized apple (13 grams of sugar) for lunch, a 20 ounce bottle of soda pop (70 grams of sugar) for an afternoon beverage, and a cup of chocolate ice cream (17 grams of sugar) during your favorite sitcom in the evening. You are taking in about 604 calories (151 grams of sugar x four calories per gram of sugar) of sugar-containing food per day without even trying. About half of those sugar carbohydrates are fructose (about 75 grams of fructose). It is actually a bit more than half because high fructose corn syrup is 55% fructose, and many fruits contain more fructose than glucose. Of note, the excess glucose accompanying the fructose can be processed by the liver and body without causing any of the chemical changes we are discussing.

Your liver can only convert about 12-18 grams of the fructose to glucose in a single day (12-15 per female, 15-18 per male). The average daily consumption of fructose in America in 1900 was 15 grams per person per day. A century later that number has risen to 90 grams per person per day. The excess fructose becomes a problem for the liver and it must process it in a different chemical pathway. Because the liver is receiving excess fructose from the intestine on a daily basis, your body undergoes a metabolic transformation within a few weeks if this becomes your dietary habit. The body's good cholesterol (HDL cholesterol) begins to fall (one of the five components of the metabolic syndrome). This cholesterol is the protective cholesterol that guards your blood vessels from forming plaque buildup on their walls. In turn, that keeps you from developing heart disease, strokes, high blood pressure and the like.

The next thing that happens is that your bad cholesterols (LDL cholesterol and VLDL cholesterol) begin to rise. These cholesterols are the fats in the bloodstream that directly contribute to the buildup of clogging fat in your blood vessels. This is just the opposite effect of the HDL cholesterol. While these are not components of the metabolic syndrome, they are signals to your physician that something is wrong. Elevations of these blood fats are associated with heart and other blood vessel diseases.

If this isn't bad enough, your serum triglyceride (another type of fat in the blood that leads to blood vessel disease when present in chronic excess) level begins to rise just a few weeks later (another component of the metabolic syndrome). The importance of the rise of this fat is detrimental in several ways. It leads to overall weight gain, accumulation of belly fat (another one of the five components of the metabolic syndrome), emergence of a fatty liver, and increased risk of heart disease over time. Really high blood levels of triglycerides can inflame the pancreas so severely that it can lead directly to your death.

Let us assume for a moment that you are a health-conscious person and work out regularly. You seem to keep your weight under control because of your increased metabolic activity from regular exercise. But you are frustrated because you just can't seem to lose weight. The fat seems to hang on your mid section. Your spare tire just won't disappear. You believe you are eating fairly healthy but can do better so you trade in your evening chocolate ice cream for a banana (14 grams of sugar versus 17 grams in the ice cream), and you trade in your fruit popup for a one cup bowl of Raisin Nut Bran cereal (27 grams of sugar versus 19 grams in the popup) for your breakfast. What is going on? You may think that you are eating healthier because you have traded in your processed food for more natural foods (fruits), but you have actually lost ground in the sugar grams department. This is one of the dilemmas facing many Americans who believe they are eating better than those who consume the sugar-laden, processed foods found in the aisles of the supermarket. Unfortunately, both are consuming too many fructose sugars chronically. The long-term consequences have already led to decreased HDL cholesterol, elevated LDL and VLDL cholesterol, elevated blood triglycerides and abdominal obesity.

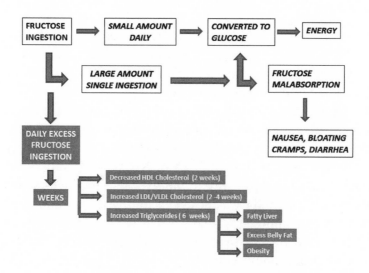

As you continue to consume excess fructose in your diet over several months your serum uric acid begins to rise. Stop right there. That is a mouthful. You weren't sure what triglyceride was and now I hit you with uric acid. Before we move forward let me help you understand the importance of this acid. As I mentioned at the outset of the chapter, Benjamin Franklin talked about apples and health. Did you know that he died from gout? Gout is a disease caused by excess uric acid in the blood stream that eventually leads to arthritis, especially in the big toe. It can affect other joints as well and it also causes kidney stones and loss of kidney function.

The cell is the basic building block of plants and animals. Every cell contains genetic material called deoxyribonucleic acid (DNA) and ribonucleic acid (RNA). These substances contain the genetic code that allows the cell to reproduce itself and produce the proteins, fats and carbohydrates essential to maintain body function. When you eat foods containing large quantities of DNA and RNA (such as some vegetables, meats, and organ foods such as brain, liver, kidney and pancreas), the body breaks down much of that genetic material and converts the waste into uric acid. Additionally, your own body has cells that die every day. Those cells need to be disposed of so the body recycles many of their parts and gets rid of the waste by the liver and kidneys. Some of that broken down material ends up as uric acid.

One of the metabolic effects of months of excess ingestion of fructose is the rise in serum uric acid. You may now say to yourself, "Where is the DNA or RNA?" Interestingly, fructose does not contain DNA or RNA, but it still stimulates a metabolic pathway in the liver that produces serum uric acid. The body was designed to digest incoming food sources containing DNA and RNA as well as processing the nucleic acid for our own dying cells. But, excess fructose overloads the body with excess uric acid production. The liver converts some of the surplus fructose into uric acid. As you learned earlier, fructose was also converted to triglyceride, and "bad" LDL and VLDL cholesterol.

It is important to note that we can also overload the body with excess uric acid production caused by genetic abnormalities of uric acid metabolism, as well as excess consumption of foods rich in DNA and RNA (eating liver, kidney or other organ foods regularly). Additionally, beer is metabolized in a fashion that leads to excess uric acid production. Beer drinkers have an increased prevalence of gout compared with drinkers of other forms of alcohol and non-drinkers of alcohol.

The deleterious effects of elevated uric acid are quite variable. While many individuals may suffer from an attack of gouty arthritis or passage of a kidney stone (like Benjamin Franklin often did in his senior years), most of us will suffer from a more insidious complication of elevated serum uric acid levels. Studies show that elevated serum uric acid levels cause blood vessel narrowing by lowering blood nitric oxide levels and increasing angiotensin levels. My goal here is not to turn you into science experts when I bring up complicated names like angiotensin and nitric oxide. But, these substances are merely the identified target chemicals that uric acid acts upon to raise your blood pressure when blood uric acid levels are persistently elevated. Both of these effects are reversible by lowering serum uric acid levels back into a normal range.

Chronically elevated serum uric acid levels, independent of the cause, lead to kidney damage, decreased sodium (salt) excretion in the urine and subsequent fluid retention. All of these effects lead directly to high blood pressure.

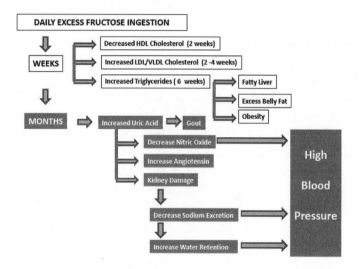

High blood pressure is another one of the components of the metabolic syndrome. In fact, we are now up to four of the five components of the metabolic syndrome, and we have only been indulging our sweet tooth for a few months with excess fructose.

What if the process of excess daily fructose intake continues for a few years? We continue to gain a belly of fat; our blood pressure continues to rise; our kidney function worsens; our liver begins to feel the strain of all the fat being deposited in it; and our blood vessels are slowly building up with deadly plaque that will lead to premature heart disease, kidney failure or stroke. But the process continues. Our body now develops a resistance to insulin and we develop type II diabetes (the fifth component of the metabolic syndrome). This is the type of diabetes that is not due to a shortage of insulin. That is type I diabetes. If we have type II diabetes, weight loss and discontinuation of all fructose in the diet will often lead to a reversal of the diabetes.

Those of you who suffer from type II diabetes, and are on medications to treat this disease, should seek medical advice if and when you reduce your fructose intake. You may require less medication as you lose weight, reduce your insulin resistance and normalize your blood sugar levels. You could suffer from very low blood sugar levels if your medication dose is not adjusted during this process, and you could suffer significant medical consequences because of the effects of low blood sugar. These can include: weakness, coldness, fatigue, light-headedness, and clammy skin, loss of consciousness, seizures, and even death. Do not take this issue lightly, and do not try to make medication adjustments without your physician's assistance.

Unchecked, diabetes leads to an abnormal heart rhythm called atrial fibrillation. Many people affected by this abnormal heart beat pattern will develop blood clots in the heart that then travel to the lungs, brain or other parts of the circulatory system. This can then cause a pulmonary embolism, stroke or other blood clot damage to the body. Additionally, type II diabetes leads to further weight gain, kidney damage, and heart disease.

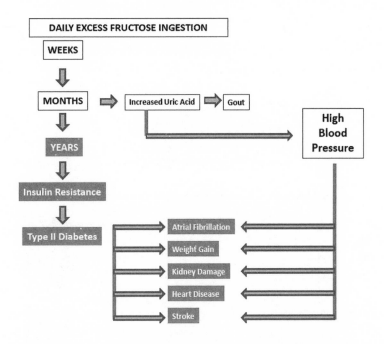

By now, I think you understand the picture. Fructose, over time, will lead to the development of every component of the metabolic syndrome directly through metabolic pathways that are turned on in the liver with continued excess consumption. What is more important, numerous medical studies involving adolescents, normal weight adults, overweight adults and research animals reveal that these processes are reversible, so long as there is no permanent damage to organs of the body like the kidneys, the heart (heart attack) or the brain (stroke). These studies show that adding excess fructose to the daily diet leads to the biochemical processes that are occurring in the liver that is causing the metabolic syndrome, removing fructose from the diet will reverse this.

There are two metabolic pathways that are utilized in the liver with excess fructose intake. The first is the conversion of the fructose to triglycerides and bad cholesterols. The other is the conversion of fructose to uric acid. The metabolic syndrome develops as a byproduct of the sustained production of these substances.

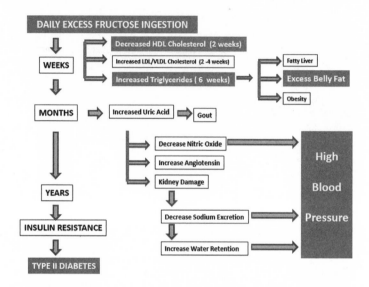

The Five Components of the Metabolic Syndrome

The present approach of the health care industry is to treat your triglyceride elevation with medications. They treat your elevated blood cholesterol with cholesterol-lowering medications. They treat your diabetes with medications. They lower your blood pressure with medications. They treat the elevated uric acid levels with more medications. In the end, you may be taking several medications for conditions that could all be treated with removal of excess daily ingestion of fructose. Now, the Food and Drug Administration is mandating that there will be a reduction of salt in the American diet implemented over the next few years. All of these medication and dietary measures may be necessary to initially manage the individual diseases, but reversing the metabolic syndrome by removing or drastically reducing the fructose intake in our diet may dramatically reduce the need for multiple lifetime medications. This is extremely important in the early years of the individual who is suffering from totally reversible aspects of the metabolic syndrome with otherwise undamaged internal organs.

While Benjamin Franklin suffered from a genetic form of excess uric acid, we will never know if eating all of those apples (which increased his uric acid levels) really helped him keep the doctor away.

Pearls

- Chronic, excessive fructose ingestion leads to the metabolic syndrome.
- Reduction of fructose intake can prevent and reverse the metabolic derangements so long as there is no permanent damage.

> "Thou seest I have more flesh than another man, and therefore more frailty." *William Shakespeare*

Chapter 12

The Fructose-Fat Connection

H ow many times have you heard someone say, "I can't lose a pound, no matter what I do?" I hear that complaint from my patients every day in my clinic. They tell me that they have altered their diets dramatically. They have tried various popularized nutrition plans, and the weight lost during their vigorous interventions promptly returns with a vengeance as soon as they relax their dietary restraints.

Why do so many Americans struggle to control their weight? One answer lies in fructose and fructose metabolism. As our consumption of fructose has increased, so has our weight. At the beginning of the twentieth century we consumed only 15 grams of fructose per day. Very few of us were overweight. As the century progressed we increased our fructose intake but maintained our weight until the introduction of high fructose corn syrup in the 1980's. Because this dramatically decreased the cost of sweetening the American diet, fructose consumption exploded in the Western diet. So did our waistlines. Not only did adults begin to bulge, so did our children. Initially, the attacks against weight gain across our land were directed toward high fructose corn syrup (HFCS) as we were now consuming over 90 grams of fructose per day, and the epidemiologic data showed a strong association between rising consumption of HFCS and the obesity epidemic developing in America. Many public school policies were examined, and this led to the removal of soda pop vending machines from lunch room cafeterias. This did not solve the problem.

As more data has been gathered in the last decade, it is now clear that the culprit for the significant weight gain in America is fructose, not just HFCS. Fructose consumption has increased primarily because of increased consumption of high fructose corn syrup, but fruit, fruit juice, honey and other sources of fructose are just as culpable. Average consumption of apples now approaches 50 pounds per person per year. Soda pop now tops 50 gallons per person, per year. The average consumption of fruit juice now tops 11 gallons per person, per year. And on and on and on.

So, what's the big deal about fructose and increasing body fat? Well, as I pointed out in the chapter about the metabolic syndrome, it takes only a few weeks of heavy consumption of fructose to cause the liver to begin to shunt fructose into a metabolic pathway that leads to triglyceride formation, rather than energy production. The effect of this process is that fructose conversion to triglyceride starts a process where belly fat now starts to grow, fatty liver formation leads to a worsening inflammation in the liver and total body weight begins to rise.

Regular excess intake of beer leads to the well known "beer belly" and it develops through the same metabolic pathway. This belly fat deposition is not necessarily the case with overeating from other sugars. The individual response to excess eating of other food products leads to global obesity of the body, while fructose overload specifically targets the abdominal cavity and liver.

What is worse is that even if you now decrease your calorie intake, your fat intake or even your fructose intake, most of the fructose you are consuming is still converted into triglyceride. This is because the enzyme pathway in the liver that is feeding this fat factory now has preferential control over fructose. Even if we are consuming fewer calories than our body needs so that we can reduce our total body weight, the fructose continues to be converted to triglyceride.

The end result is that our bellies refuse to get smaller, even if our total weight has decreased. When you are walking through your local shopping mall, you will see young people who are not necessarily overweight, but who have a spare tire hanging over the top of their designer jeans. Yet, their bodies otherwise are relatively lean. This is because the metabolic syndrome is in play with the conversion of fructose to triglyceride that is then being deposited in the belly fat of these adolescents. This phenomenon is the so called "muffin top" that is hanging over the jeans of many teenagers with otherwise well-proportioned bodies. As we age, we see more and more people affected by so-called beer bellies and loss of waistlines, in spite of the lack of significant beer consumption. It is because of this same problem.

What is the solution to this vicious cycle? You can't just reduce fructose intake to stop or reverse this process. You need to **restrict your diet to a total fructose fast for a few weeks to shut down the conversion of fructose to triglyceride, "bad" LDL/VLDL cholesterol and fructose to uric acid enzyme pathways by the liver**. It takes two to three weeks to accomplish this process. While you are doing this you will go through a physical withdrawal from fructose that can be rather difficult. First of all, fructose is included in most processed foods today. Additionally, honey, fruits, fruit juices, foods containing high fructose corn syrup or table sugar, and some vegetables contain significant quantities of fructose. Trying to avoid all of these fructose sources can be daunting while you are trying to shut down this fat-forming factory in the liver.

Before I proceeded to write this chapter, I challenged myself, my spouse, my sister and several coworkers to go through this process to see how we would do. While weight loss came easier for some than others, the withdrawal from fructose was rather dramatic in nearly all of us. Additionally, finding foods that would satiate our appetites was also a challenge. After a few weeks though, our waistlines began to shrink and some us of were on our way to clothes sizes that we had not been able to wear for the past few years. Once we got through the withdrawal period, we no longer had an insatiable hunger for sweets. In fact, many could take or leave them without any immediate relapse to our old ways of high fructose consumption. What's more, if we did find ourselves craving the sugar again by cranking the fat enzyme factory back into gear, all we had to do was go through another two to three week fast from fructose to shut it down again. Easier said than done, but at least we were able to shut down the metabolic syndrome developing in our body.

It is amazing just how big the obesity situation in America has become in the past twenty-five years. From the 1960s until 1980 the obesity rate was fairly flat at 13-15% of Americans. But the next decade saw a rapid rise in obesity to 23% by 1994. The rate continued to climb so that by 2007 the number topped 27% of the adult population. At the same time, those considered overweight have dramatically increased so that two-thirds of the population in the United States is considered overweight or obese. Additionally, nearly four million Americans now weigh over 300 pounds and 400,000 individuals weigh over 400 pounds.

The introduction of high fructose corn syrup into our diet parallels the weight explosion in America. But, as I pointed out earlier, fructose consumption is the real culprit. High fructose corn syrup allowed sweets of all types to become inexpensive, and consumption of this sugar exploded along with our waistlines.

Children and adolescents have also been affected by the increased consumption of inexpensive sugar. Prior to the introduction of high fructose corn syrup into our diet, approximately 6% of youth across all ages were obese. That number for all ages of children and young adults has steadily increased since the 1980s to the present level of 12% for children, ages 2-5 years; and, 18% for those ages 6-19 years. During the same time that Americans have gotten larger, the number of individuals developing high blood pressure, gout, type II diabetes, gallbladder disease, heart disease, kidney disease, cancer associated with obesity (breast, esophagus and colon), and associated deaths has increased as well. Obesity-related death is now estimated at 400,000 people per year; and treating obesity-related diseases accounts for up to 12% of our health care costs in America, approaching 118 billion dollars per year.

Fructose is at the heart and waistline of this epidemic. While people are consuming more calories in general, fructose alters our metabolism and that directly leads to waistline obesity and the diseases of the metabolic syndrome that follow. Unless we change our eating habits, the problem will only get worse. The youth of America will soon be adults, and there is no data to suggest that they will not add to the obesity rate already rising in the adult population. Along with waistline obesity and its associated diseases, the costs to our society in health care costs will grow as well. Additionally, productivity of America's workforce will be plagued by lost work due to health-related testing, the massive cost of medical and surgical treatment (some patients suffering from all components of the metabolic syndrome may be taking five or more medications per day), absenteeism for illnesses related to the diseases developing in young people related to the metabolic syndrome, and premature death because of this preventable epidemic. The effects are staggering. The sooner we all understand the devastating affects of fructose on our health, the sooner we can reverse the processes with dietary changes.

Pearls

- Chronic, excess fructose ingestion leads to abdominal (central) obesity.
- Obesity is now an epidemic problem in America.
- Restricting your diet to a total fructose fast for a few weeks will shut down the conversion of fructose that would otherwise perpetuate the metabolic syndrome.

"The task of the modern educator is not to cut down jungles, but to irrigate deserts." *C. S. Lewis*

Chapter 13

Glucose and Other Sugars are Different

Fructose is a sugar with unique properties. It is far sweeter than other sugars. This makes it quite appealing to our taste buds. As I explained in an earlier chapter, there is altered brain signaling by fructose through the hormone leptin, which leads to overeating because the brain has been tricked into thinking not enough food has been eaten. Other sugars do not cause us to crave them like fructose because they do not alter leptin sensitivity. You learned that **the driving force behind turning on the metabolic syndrome is the chronic, excess ingestion of fructose**.

Other sugars found in our food supply are not the culprits of this problem. They may taste good, but not overly so. They may add calories to our diet, but not overly so. And, they could lead to weight gain if we eat them to excess regularly, but not overly so. **They do not cause the metabolic syndrome in animal studies or humans. Fructose is the only sugar that is known to do this**.

What is even more important, the other sugars do not lead to any known diseases that are now directly linked to continued, excess ingestion of fructose. While other sugars are processed in various metabolic compartments in the body (brain, liver, kidneys, muscles, etc.) fructose is processed only by the liver. When we consume glucose (simple sugar; starch of potatoes or rice) all cells in the human body can directly use this sugar as a form of energy that allows muscles to contract, nerve cells to fire, generate body heat, read this book, etc. **Most importantly, glucose does not generate the metabolic syndrome in animal or human studies**.

Likewise, galactose (the sugar found in milk that is chemically connected to a glucose molecule to form lactose or milk sugar) is metabolized by the body and is converted to glucose. It can then be used for energy or stored for future energy needs in the form of glycogen (the stored form of glucose; this occurs in muscles and liver). Galactose is thought to have some direct benefit to nerve and kidney cells, and it prevents cataracts. The majority of this sugar is converted to glucose by the liver. The glucose can then be used in the production of energy by our body or stored as glycogen. **Galactose excess, like excess consumption of glucose, does not produce the metabolic syndrome.**

Other sugars found in nature are of minimal importance in the nutrition of humans. Most are not digestible in our enzyme systems and are fermented by colonic bacteria. We may experience symptoms of that fermentation process as the bacteria generate intestinal gas. Many of us may feel abdominal bloating, nausea, cramping, flatulence and diarrhea in some cases.

When fructose is ingested it is metabolized only by the liver. When ingested in small quantities, the liver converts it to glucose. The body handles this glucose in the manner outlined earlier in this chapter. Excess glucose is stored in the body as glycogen. If all the glycogen storage sites are filled, excess glucose is converted to body fat. If the body is in need of glucose to supply energy for vital functions, it is transported by the bloodstream to the point where cells need to put it to use. This small ingestion and glucose conversion has no deleterious effect on the body.

Suppose that you had been consuming only a small amount of fructose on a daily basis, but today you went to the office picnic where you pigged out on fruit salad, watermelon, cookies, sugar-sweetened iced tea, cake, and ice cream, consuming 200 grams of fructose. Besides feeling a little sick to your stomach with fructose malabsorption when you get home, your liver has to figure out what to do with all that fructose. If it is a one-time event, the body will convert as much of it to glucose that the enzyme pathway allows; the excess does not activate the metabolic syndrome. This only occurs with persistent overloading of the liver with fructose. The surplus fructose is shunted into two different metabolism pathways. The first is the pathway that leads to the production of uric acid, the substance that leads to gout, high blood pressure, and kidney disease. The second is the pathway that leads to the production of fatty acids, LDL/VLDL cholesterol (bad cholesterol) and triglycerides. These pathway products cause fatty liver disease, cirrhosis of the liver, liver failure, abdominal obesity, insulin resistance, type II diabetes, esophageal reflux disease, cancer of the colon, breast, and esophagus, heart disease, and premature death. The longer you consume daily, excess fructose (regardless of its source) the more tissue damage occurs throughout the body.

The other sugars found in our diet do not stimulate either of these metabolic pathways in the liver. The ongoing stimulation of these pathways by fructose leads to the metabolic syndrome that I describe in chapters 10 and 11. While eating too much sugar other than fructose can lead to obesity because of excess calories in relationship to the body's energy needs, it does not lead to the activation of these deleterious metabolic pathways.

Obesity Effects

In describing the metabolic syndrome, I did not spend much time discussing all of the specific diseases in those chapters. When we chronically ingest large quantities of fructose, two enzymes are turned on in the liver cells that convert fructose to a type of fat called triglyceride. This fat is then deposited in the abdominal cavity and the liver. The excess abdominal fat is what is called central obesity. Central obesity places excess pressure on the diaphragm especially after a large meal. The abdominal cavity is a positive pressure system in relation to the atmosphere outside the body. Meanwhile the chest cavity is a negative pressure system compared to the atmosphere outside the body. After a meal, excess pressure in the abdomen created by the food placed in the stomach and the obese abdomen place undue pressure on the diaphragm. This causes stretching of the opening of the diaphragm where the esophagus passes from the chest into the abdomen. The larger the abdomen becomes from triglyceride production from excess fructose, the more sustained is the pressure on the diaphragm. The chronic, daily stretching of this opening causes a hernia to form. This hernia is named a hiatus hernia because the opening is called the diaphragm hiatus. As pressure is repeatedly transmitted through the diaphragm and the hernia enlarges, the sphincter protecting the esophagus from the stomach is broken down. Then, when we eat specific trigger foods, beverages, spices or herbs, we regurgitate our gastric contents from the stomach into the esophagus. This is known as gastroesophageal reflux disease (GERD). The consequences of longstanding GERD can include adult-onset asthma, chronic cough, aspiration pneumonias, interstitial fibrosis (scarring) of the lung, respiratory failure, throat cancer, loss of enamel from your teeth and esophageal cancer. Additionally, snoring, forms of sleep apnea, sinus and ear problems occur in some individuals affected by chronic GERD.

Reflux-induced esophageal cancer is the fastest rising cancer in America, and it is strongly associated with central obesity. The incidence of esophageal cancer has risen over 600% in the last 30 years. Central obesity has dramatically increased in all age groups in that same time period. It is interesting to note that this type of obesity is primarily caused by chronic, excess ingestion of fructose.

Fatty Liver Effect

Fatty liver disease has several causes, but the cause that has taken us the longest time to understand is excess fructose ingestion. Other sugars are not known to cause fatty liver disease. In my lifetime as a gastrointestinal physician I have seen the incidence of fatty liver move from obscurity to the leading cause of liver disease in America. While essential fatty acid deficiency clearly can cause fatty liver disease (see my previous book: *42 Days to a New Life*), it is also now clear that chronic, excess fructose ingestion leads to triglyceride production. These triglycerides (fats) are then deposited in the liver as well as the abdominal cavity (see above).

It is unclear why some individuals with fatty liver will not suffer significant liver damage. For those that do, my feeling is that it is a combination of excess inflammatory fat (linoleic acid, also known as omega-6 fatty acid), consumption of trans fats (highly inflammatory), and a shortage of anti-inflammatory fat (alpha linolenic acid, also known as omega-3 fatty acid) in our diet in the presence of the fatty liver from chronic fructose ingestion that ignites the inflammatory process in the liver. We are now seeing fatty liver disease in the youth of America. The Mayo Clinic recently published data concerning their fatty liver disease experience where they had to perform liver transplantations on children who had developed fatty liver disease. I have also seen adolescents with advanced liver disease because of this process.

Fatty liver disease may lead to cirrhosis of the liver like the liver scarring seen in chronic alcoholics. The consequences of cirrhosis in this setting can be intestinal bleeding (from dilated esophageal veins called esophageal varices), excess fluid buildup in the abdominal cavity (known as ascites), confusion (known as hepatic encephalopathy), liver cancer, kidney failure, coma and death. These are amazing consequences for having that morning fruit smoothie, eating several pieces of fruit every day, drinking 2-3 glasses of fruit juice per day, eating too many cookies or candies, drinking a 20 ounce bottle of soda pop at lunch, etc., too frequently for too many years.

Many of us are suffering from excess fructose in our diet and are unaware of its consequences until we develop a medical complication of fatty liver disease or esophageal reflux disease. Once our bodies are suffering from these problems the chance for reversal of the disease-induced damage is diminished. This is especially true if we do not understand the cause: chronic, daily, excess fructose intake.

Uric Acid Effects

Consumed in chronic excess, fructose leads to elevated blood levels of a substance called uric acid. This elevated level of uric acid is called hyperuricemia. The importance of hyperuricemia is that it can lead to a disease called gout. Gout was known as the "disease of kings," and it dates back to 2640 BC in ancient Egypt. One of the most famous people of world history, Benjamin Franklin, suffered from a genetically-inherited form of gout.

Gout is an inflammatory joint disease caused by uric acid crystals becoming deposited in and around our joints. Chronic hyperuricemia is the cause of gout, and the incidence of gout has doubled in America in the past 25 years. One of the contributing factors to the rise of gout in the U.S. is that fructose intake has dramatically increased in that same time period. Fructose, in chronic excess, is metabolized by the liver to form uric acid. When enough uric acid builds up in the blood, it saturates the body and crystallizes. Once crystallized, the uric acid is highly inflammatory to tissue. When this occurs in the joint spaces we develop an intense arthritis reaction that is said to be one of the most painful, sudden-onset maladies ever experienced by patients.

While there are other causes of elevated uric acid levels, rapidly rising consumption of fructose in the western diet since the 1980s has been a major contributor to the doubling of the incidence of gout in America. Not all people with hyperuricemia will develop full blown gout. Those with chronically elevated uric acid levels place an undo pressure on the kidneys as uric acid is primarily excreted by the kidneys (two-thirds of it) while the rest is excreted by the intestine. The kidney excretion of excess uric acid leads to several problems. First, the uric acid will directly damage the kidney. This can lead to decreased kidney function, eventual kidney failure and death without dialysis or a kidney transplant. Second, the kidney damage from the uric acid leads to decreased salt excretion in the urine. This process causes fluid retention in the body's tissues and blood vessels. The excess fluid load then causes high blood pressure.

Chronic high blood pressure is now the most common disease in America affecting 67 million adults and many youth. Over time it can cause an enlarged heart with subsequent heart failure, vision damage, worsening kidney function, strokes and heart attacks, aneurysms of blood vessels, and the list goes on. Continued high blood pressure is a silent killer as we do not have many symptoms while organ damage is occurring. As you can see, this is a major misery to our health all because of satisfying our sweet tooth (or, I should say, taste buds).

Intestinal Malabsorption

Another major problem of excess intake of fructose in one sitting is fructose malabsorption. Have you ever wondered why you or a loved one will get intestinal cramping, bloating, abdominal pain and even diarrhea after eating certain foods? While many foods may cause similar symptoms for a variety of reasons, my focus at the moment is excess fructose. Our intestinal tract is designed to handle eating only a few grams of fructose at a single intake. If we exceed that threshold of fructose absorption, we will develop gastrointestinal distress. The reason for this is that the excess fructose travels from the intestine into the colon without being absorbed into the bloodstream. In the colon this sugar will be fermented by the colonic bacteria. The bacteria feast on the fructose, and the product of bacterial fermentation is the generation of gas (hydrogen, carbon dioxide, methane, etc.). As the gas generated by the bacteria builds up in the intestine, it leads to abdominal distention, bloating, cramping, pain and flatulence. Additionally, the fructose, by osmosis, will pull water into the intestine which is carried into the colon where diarrhea may ensue.

Just how much fructose is needed to cause this malabsorption problem? Several studies have been performed to address this question, but one of my favorites is from the University of Kansas. Gastrointestinal scientists performed a randomized, double-blind study on healthy young 26-year-old men who had no medical problems. The men ingested 0, 25 or 50 grams of fructose in a capsule and then answered questionnaires about the symptoms they sustained. They were unaware of what they were ingesting, as were the scientists. When they analyzed the results, the findings were amazing to say the least. With 0 grams of fructose 0/16 men had intestinal symptoms; with 25 grams 8/16 developed symptoms; and, with 50 grams of fructose 11/16 men developed malabsorption symptoms.

Grams Fructose Ingested	% Symptoms
0	0
25	50
50	68

To help put the quantity of fructose used in this study into perspective, a 12 ounce can of soda pop contains about 22 grams of fructose. It is easy to see why so many people suffer from an irritable bowel problem with today's diet containing such large quantities of fructose found in supersized drinks, Big Gulps and now the standard-sized 20 ounce soda pops. Malabsorption from fructose, whether it is from consuming excessive amounts of soda pop, several pieces of fruit per day, fruit juices, fruit smoothies, candies, cookies, muffins, most breads and cakes (the list seems endless) is directly responsible for frequent bouts of misery for millions of Americans. Yet, most do not make the connection.

Many people suffer from intestinal bloating, flatulence and intermittent diarrhea on a regular basis. While fructose malabsorption of a large, single ingestion of fructose may be causing the symptoms, a significant percentage of individuals suffer from an altered gut flora that is directly linked to excess fructose intake that causes bacteria to colonize the small intestine and produce these symptoms. This is referred to as bacterial overgrowth, and is often remedied with "probiotic" cultures of beneficial bacteria that reestablish a normal gut flora or short courses of antibiotics that are prescribed by a physician. The problem becomes cyclic however, if fructose is continually ingested in high quantities as the colonic bacteria again take up residence in the small intestine. You can see the vicious cycle that develops just because of consuming too much fructose.

Type II Diabetes

Diabetes is another disease on the rise in America over the past 25 years. Diabetes is a disorder of blood sugar (glucose) regulation. Insulin is a hormone produced in the pancreas that controls blood sugar levels. When we either do not make enough insulin (type I diabetes) or our body's cells become resistant to the effects of insulin (type II diabetes), our blood sugars become quite elevated. There are many consequences of chronically-elevated blood sugar levels. Our metabolism can be dangerously altered to the point that we can die from a buildup of toxic acids in our blood. More frequently however, we will suffer nerve damage, kidney damage, vision damage, heart disease, damage to other blood vessels and many intestinal problems, including recurrent nausea and vomiting, chronic diarrhea, gastric paralysis and premature death.

Type II diabetes now accounts for 90% of all cases of diabetes in the United States. We are witnessing children, adolescents and young adults developing diabetes at a rate never seen before. This, again, is directly and indirectly linked to chronic, excess consumption of fructose. Fructose does not directly affect insulin activity in the body. Rather, fructose stimulates uric acid (hyperuricemia) production with chronic, excess consumption. This metabolic state of hyperuricemia leads to insulin resistance in the cells of the body. The body reacts by developing central obesity, chronically elevated blood sugar levels and eventually the long-term consequences of diabetes if the process is not arrested.

The sad thing about insulin resistance is that it can be completely reversed with abstinence of fructose and aggressive weight loss. I have a patient in my practice that developed type II diabetes, morbid obesity, high blood pressure, fatty liver and elevated blood triglyceride levels in her early 20s. She was determined to take control of her rapidly-deteriorating life, as she was on several medications to treat her conditions, constantly undergoing blood tests, x-rays and the like, and spending a lot of time and money in doctor offices. When she gave up sweets of all types and lost over a hundred pounds, virtually all of her medical conditions reversed themselves. She is now off all of her medications and her metabolism has returned to normal. She is now judicious in her consumption of fructose products, and she is diligently keeping her weight under control. Her medical problems have not recurred. This is a living example of an individual who was plagued by the metabolic syndrome, all because of chronic, excess fructose consumption.

Blood Vessel Disease

The last area on which I want to focus in this chapter is blood vessel disease. The statistics for morbidity and mortality related to blood vessel disease in America are staggering. Over 1,500,000 individuals suffer heart attacks each year. Eight hundred sixty thousand deaths from cardiovascular disease were reported in 2005 (one death every 37 seconds). Additionally, 780,000 people suffer from a stroke each year, and an individual dies every 40 seconds from stroke-related complications. An additional 300,000 people die of heart failure every year. Many others suffer from blood clots in their abdominal and leg blood vessels leading to significant loss of life.

While the causes of all these blood vessel diseases are quite complicated, we know that there are specific contributors to the development of blood vessel disease that lead to suffering and death.

We have blood markers that reflect an increased risk of suffering from one of these disorders. One of those markers is the blood elevation of "bad" cholesterol (LDL cholesterol). At the same time we often see a drop in "good" cholesterol (HDL cholesterol). In the past 15 years of studies in preparation for the writing of this and my previous book, I now know of two specific reasons for which we see these cholesterol changes in the blood.

The first is the chronic ingestion of human manufactured trans fats (also known as partially hydrogenated vegetable oils, such as hydrogenated soybean oil, hydrogenated cottonseed oil, etc.). I spent several years of my medical life doing the library homework to discover the devastating effects of these highly inflammatory oils on the human body. Finland has discovered this fact as well, and in the 1970s they outlawed the presence of any trans fats in their food supply. Since that time, their country has seen a 50% reduction of heart disease. In 1950, there were 500 cardiologists practicing in America. Today, that number has increased to 21,000 heart specialists; and the demand for many more is projected based on the rising incidence of heart disease in the United States. Maybe we can learn from the Scandinavians by choosing to consume foods devoid of all trans fats in this country to stem the tide against the suffering and death incurred from cardiac diseases. That would be very meaningful healthcare reform.

The second established cause of blood vessel disease is the metabolic syndrome. As I outlined before, the primary cause of metabolic syndrome is chronic, overindulgence of fructose. Fructose can activate the metabolic syndrome in a matter of weeks of excess consumption. Our medical group recently saw this process in play in a 15-year-old young man who has the metabolic syndrome. He was a survivor of a heart attack and was in our office for treatment of his fatty liver. His body was paying the price of unchecked metabolic syndrome caused by excessive fructose intake. And, at a very young age.

I find it fascinating that the U.S. Government strongly recommended increasing daily fruit consumption in November 2009 during the heated congressional debates over healthcare reform. At the same time, they were contemplating taxation of the soda pop industry to curtail fructose consumption. This was all occurring while the federal government was subsidizing the corn crop industry so that they can manufacture more high fructose corn syrup. Perhaps they should encourage farmers to convert their crops from corn to flax, mandate the curtailment of all manufactured trans fats in our food supply and recommend manufacturers markedly reduce fructose inclusion in food products. This could be accomplished through the use of sucralose or other artificial sweeteners (more on this in a later chapter), the use of glucose polymers as sweeteners (they don't cause these problems), and most importantly, the education of our society about the truth relating to all of this information. These kinds of real healthcare reforms would save Americans billions of dollars in health care costs, lost productivity, and immeasurable suffering from medical conditions. And, hundreds of thousands, if not millions of lives might be spared annually if these real preventative measures were implemented. All of these changes can be implemented by each one of us individually making educated choices at the supermarket, restaurants and our dining tables.

Pearls

- Glucose and other sugars do not cause the metabolic syndrome.
- Only chronic, excess fructose intake causes the metabolic syndrome.
- Obesity, fatty liver disease, gout, high blood pressure, intestinal malabsorption, type II diabetes and blood vessel disease all occur from excess fructose in the diet.

"What you leave behind is not what is engraved in stone monuments, but what is woven into the lives of others." *Pericles*

Chapter 14

Reversing the Fructose Effect

I magine for a moment you are floating down the Niagara River from Lake Erie to Lake Ontario in a canoe heading straight toward the powerful Niagara Falls. While the rare individual may survive the initial 70 foot drop, the next 100 feet is a bumpy fall over a cascade of boulders that kills nearly everyone unless they have made the journey in a heavily constructed barrel. But you are just sitting in your canoe with little or no real protection from the drop ahead of you. At some point, as you near the precipice of the falls, you will reach a point of no return. Either you turn your canoe around, fight the current, and escape the drop; or you plunge over the falls toward trauma and death. And nobody has ever paddled back up the falls.

In medicine I face similar dilemmas daily as I counsel patients about the long-term effects of continuing unhealthy life choices. The natural history of many diseases has been established. For example, the natural history of surviving a chronic hepatitis C infection averages 30-40 years. Yet, that is only the mean (the midpoint average of all survivors from the quickest death to the longest survivor) life expectancy after acquiring the infection. I have seen patients live with the virus infecting their liver for 55 years with little damage, while others have succumbed to the disease in less than a decade.

The same wide variation is seen in many other medical situations. Chronic AIDS virus infection, chronic alcohol abuse, chronic addictive drug use, chronic cigarette or marijuana smoking, chronic high blood pressure that has not been controlled, chronic elevation of blood sugar that has not been controlled and chronic trans fat ingestion are just a few of those situations.

Chronic, excess fructose ingestion is the new canoe floating down the river toward the falls. As I pointed out in Chapter 11 concerning fructose and the metabolic syndrome, we see metabolic changes start to occur in our bodies as early as two weeks into chronic, excess ingestion. We already have begun our float toward the falls. As more and more of the metabolic changes develop, there is a point where our body will go over the falls. Once that occurs our bodies are unable to reverse the damage caused by all the metabolic changes that have occurred by chronic, excess fructose ingestion.

I have had many patients at various stages of liver damage from fructose ingestion who were highly motivated to change their diets and reverse the liver scarring. Others have not been so inspired, and they have progressed to cirrhosis at very young ages. Kidney damage, blood vessel disease, liver disease, inflammatory arthritis from gout, end organ damage from chronic high blood pressure and diabetes, chronic atrial fibrillation (an irregular heart rhythm) arising from chronic insulin resistance and type II diabetes and cancers associated with obesity all have different natural histories. The problem is that at some point many of the disease processes are progressing in our body simultaneously, and they cannot be reversed. The canoe cannot be turned around.

You may have developed high blood pressure, elevated LDL (bad) cholesterol, elevated blood triglycerides, chronically elevated uric acid levels, mild diabetes, etc. Your physician will have placed you on several new medications to treat your blood pressure, abnormal heart rhythm or elevated blood chemistries. But if you could just stop consuming this deadly sugar, many of the metabolic changes would dramatically improve without medications. If end organ damage is mild, our bodies have an amazing ability to heal. Individuals with more advanced disease states will be less fortunate.

I learned from the trans fat and omega-3 fatty acid literature that even significant heart disease can be reversed just by aggressively changing our diet. Likewise, we cannot reverse cirrhosis of the liver, but in many instances we can stop progression and reverse scarring up to the final point of cirrhosis. It requires a drastic change in our lifestyle, and the self-discipline to stay the course. Otherwise, the canoe will just turn back toward the falls, and the same disaster awaits.

If we continue with the Niagara Falls illustration a bit further, we would never get in the river above the falls in the first place if we knew what was ahead of us as we paddled down stream. Either we would get out of the water upstream and carry our canoe around the falls where we could safely reenter the river, or we would find an alternate path to travel altogether. Similarly, if we are already traveling down the metabolic syndrome river, we need to get out of the water before it is too late. For most of us (over 65% of the U.S. population), not getting in the river is not an option. We are already in the metabolic syndrome river. For the majority of us who are already floating toward the cascading falls, we need to eliminate fructose from our diet, lose weight and restore our health before irreversible end-organ damage has carried us to chronic suffering and premature death.

Studies are already emerging in the medical literature where processes that have developed in patients with early metabolic syndrome are completely reversible with aggressive changes of the high fructose lifestyle. The same is true

in reversing the inflammatory damage from chronic ingestion of trans fat and in the deficiency of omega-3 fatty acid
in our diet as my previous book discusses at length.

Little data is yet available in the literature to pass on to
you about beginning the destructive process from chronic
excess consumption of fructose in people who have developed irreversible liver, kidney, heart, blood vessel or joint
damage. But, common sense tells me that we should stop
paddling toward the waterfalls. We should get out of the
"metabolic syndrome" river and stay out. Staying in the
mode of excess fructose ingestion is not allowing the body
to reverse the destructive course you are on, regardless of
the degree of damage your body has suffered. The metabolic
syndrome has been destroying the health of America only
for the past 30 years, and science began teaching us that it is
caused by chronic fructose excess in our diet fairly recently.
Consequently, there is no long-term information concerning
the improvement that might occur in those of us who have
already gone over the falls of irreversible end organ damage.
The majority of us are already in the metabolic syndrome
river. The sooner we get out of the water, the sooner we can
allow our bodies to initiate a healing process, or at least stop
advancing our diseases that we already suffer from.

When we look at the need for healthcare reform in this
country, you can easily see that avoiding the metabolic
syndrome river that leads our bodies to destruction over
the waterfalls by avoiding excess fructose ingestion in our
diet is far less expensive than treating the multiple chronic
conditions that develop by doing otherwise. The expensive
medications, numerous bills from doctor visits, hospitaliza-
tions and laboratory testing, lost revenue from missed work
because of disability, disease care management, and the like,
are huge financial burdens rapidly developing in America.

We learned from the Trans fat ban in Finland that heart
disease could decrease by 50% in just 25 years. This inter-

vention reduced the cost of healthcare for that country in untold amounts, let alone the decreased suffering and death associated with heart disease. The same avoidance of trans fats along with dramatic reduction of daily excess fructose ingestion, and increased daily intake of omega-3 fatty acids in our diet, could dramatically reduce the cost of healthcare and improve the quality of our lives in the United States. The power to make these dietary changes rests solely with each of us. It requires personal education about the consequences of doing otherwise, the desire to live a long, healthy life, and the self discipline to make the necessary dietary changes.

Pearls

- The metabolic consequences of chronic, excess fructose ingestion are reversible to a point.

- Once there is end organ damage from the metabolic syndrome, much of that destruction is not reversible.

"A man's errors are his portals of discovery."
James Joyce

Chapter 15

The Glycemic Index Fallacy

Trying to convince someone about facts that contradict the medical myth can be a daunting challenge. Many of these myths, if believed by individuals, actually may be detrimental to your health. One example of a medical myth that I deal with daily is the continued belief by many that you should not eat seeds, nuts or popcorn if you have diverticulosis in your colon. The medical condition is a disorder of the colon where you have developed pockets, or outpouchings, in the bowel lining caused by a long period of low fiber intake in your diet. Dating back to the 1950s patients who were identified with this malady were advised not to eat seeds, nuts or popcorn. If you develop inflammation of your diverticulosis you could suffer from pain in the abdomen, intestinal bleeding, infection in a diverticulum and even perforation of the bowel wall. A severe case could lead to peritonitis or death. During times of inflammation of a diverticulum all forms of fiber should be avoided, including your seeds, nuts or popcorn. However, in the individual who is not suffering from any of these complications, consumption of these fiber sources are actually beneficial to the bowel. Interestingly, the only known cause of colon inflammation in patients with diverticulosis is the use of nonsteroidal anti-inflammatory medications such as ibuprofen, naproxen, aspirin, etc. There has never been a published case of a seed, nut or popcorn kernel found in a pathology specimen from an individual who needed surgery for a complication of their diverticulosis.

The point of this chapter is not to site a litany of medical myths, but to dispel some confusion concerning the ingestion of fructose as it relates to blood sugar levels, insulin resistance and diabetes. When we consume various forms of sugar, the intestine transports some of them into the bloodstream where they are carried to the liver for further processing. As I mentioned in an earlier chapter, glucose is the primary blood sugar. A small amount of transported fructose is converted by the liver into glucose. Galactose is also converted to glucose. Most of the other ingested sugars are carried into the colon where bacteria digest them.

As the liver processes the blood sugar (glucose) coming in from the intestine, our blood sugar levels begin to rise and we develop hyperglycemia (elevated blood sugar). Alternatively, between meals our body consumes the blood sugar for energy needs and our blood sugar begins to fall. This is called hypoglycemia. Glycemia only refers to blood sugar or glucose levels. Other forms of sugars are not measured by your physician because nearly all circulating sugar in our bloodstream is glucose, and the other sugars are not regulated by insulin. Insulin is a hormone manufactured in the pancreas that acts to regulate blood levels of glucose. It has no effect on fructose, galactose (milk sugar), sugar alcohols, etc. As blood glucose levels rise, insulin is released by the pancreas to lower this sugar level. If the blood glucose level falls, the insulin levels decrease so that the blood sugar levels can rise again. Stored glucose, in the form of glycogen in the liver and muscle cells, are mobilized to restore blood sugar levels.

While the fine-tuning controls of blood glucose levels are more intricate than what I have just outlined, this understanding will help you understand the glycemic index. The glycemic index is a number ranking system of foods that was developed by a team of medical research scientists in the 1970s that predicts how rapidly blood glucose levels will rise if you eat a particular food. A single serving of glucose (one teaspoonful) was given an arbitrary score of 100, and other foods are assigned a glycemic index number relative to how much that food or beverage raises your blood glucose compared to pure glucose ingestion.

Table 1. Glycemic Index of Some Common Foods Compared with Grams of Fructose per Serving

Food Product	Glycemic Index	Gms Fructose/Serving
Glucose	100	0.00 grams
Fructose	22	4.00 grams
Table Sugar	64	2.00 grams
Apple	38	10.74 grams
Cherries	22	7.41 grams
Cheerios Cereal	74	0.50 grams
Frosted Flakes Cereal	55	6.00 grams
Sourdough Bread	54	0.00 grams
Whole Wheat Bread	68	1.30 grams
Soda Pop	65	20.20 grams
Whole Milk	30	0.00 grams
White Mashed Potato	70	0.00 grams
Sweet Potato	52	3.00 grams
Beef Steak	0	0.00 grams
Salmon Steak	0	0.00 grams
Chicken Breast	0	0.00 grams

For example, if you eat a starchy food such as rice or a white potato, your blood glucose level will rise quickly;

eating protein such as a piece of chicken will cause it to rise much more slowly. These starchy foods are assigned to a high glycemic index while the chicken is assigned a much lower number. It can be seen from some of the above-listed foods that foods and beverages that are very high in fructose have a low glycemic index versus meats, which do not have any type of sugar present. Yet, these products will lead to the metabolic syndrome and the many diseases that follow if they are ingested in excess of the liver's ability to convert the fructose to glucose.

It only takes about 20 to 30 grams of fructose per day in most people to start up the biochemical processes which will lead to the metabolic syndrome. Other food products have no fructose, yet have a high glycemic index and these foods do not cause the metabolic syndrome.

The glycemic index was developed for individuals who are suffering from diabetes (chronically elevated blood sugar levels) so that they could better control their blood sugar levels with selections of low glycemic index foods. Diabetes can occur because of insulin deficiency or insulin resistance. Insulin deficiency is called type I diabetes and usually develops in childhood. All of these individuals need to inject insulin regularly in order to control their blood sugar levels. Insulin resistance is called type II diabetes. This occurs because of chronic, excess fructose ingestion and obesity.

Individuals with either type of diabetes have been taught to avoid high glycemic index foods in order to prevent a rapid rise in blood glucose levels. Because sugars such as fructose do not cause our blood glucose levels to rise (fructose has a low glycemic index), physicians began to recommend the use of fructose in the diet of individuals suffering from diabetes. In theory it sounded great, but as I discussed earlier, chronic, excess fructose ingestion leads to insulin resistance and type II diabetes. By following these recommendations, the fructose consumption was actually contributing to the worsening of diabetes in these individuals.

Additionally, individuals who do not suffer from diabetes, but work diligently with dietary management in avoiding high starch foods that typically have a high glycemic index can develop insulin resistance and type II diabetes if they have switched to more natural, high fructose foods and beverages as alternative energy sources. They may consume a fruit smoothie for breakfast, drink fruit juices as snacks, enjoy fruit at lunch, etc. and by the end of the day they have ingested dozens of grams of fructose. They believe that they have been consuming very healthy, low glycemic index foods, and they are improving their overall health with a natural diet. They are avoiding table sugar, sweets and high fructose corn syrup, and starchy foods with a high glycemic index; and, they are eating healthy, natural foods that are much better for them. Even the federal government made a strong push for children to consume more fresh fruit in November 2009.

Yet, science says otherwise. While the chemistry of fructose metabolism does not have a high glycemic index, it leads to insulin resistance, obesity in susceptible individuals and type II diabetes. We have now seen an epidemic of these problems develop over the past 25 years in America. While increased ingestion of the combinations of table sugar (50% fructose) and high fructose corn syrup (typically 55% fructose) has been documented in that time period, our ingestion of fructose from fruit, fruit juices, fruit smoothies (as noted before, there are even "fast-food" chains that specialize in fruit smoothies at most malls in America today) and the like has skyrocketed. It all contributes to insulin resistance, obesity, and type II diabetes.

Nature designed it so that we could consume fructose just a few weeks out of the year. Scientific advancements in the 19th and 20th centuries brought us the canning process, refrigeration, freezing, pasteurization, nitrogen storage, rapid transport of commodities, radiation treatment of foods, seed hybridization, etc. Because of these technologic advancements we can now consume fruits and their products 24/7, 365 days a year. We eat kiwi fruit from New Zealand, pineapple from the Philippines, tomatoes from Guatemala, and on and on and on. In the past, we consumed fresh fruit from our own gardens and orchards or from the local market (if we were financially well off) for the few days of the year that it was "in season", but now we can eat our favorite fruit every day of the year. The human body was not designed metabolically to process the daily deluge of high fructose consumption. In a very short period of time, the metabolic syndrome turns on, insulin resistance develops, and we are on our way to developing type II diabetes.

While diabetics may benefit from utilizing the glycemic index to choose foods that will not cause wide swings in their blood sugar levels, substituting food high in fructose (it has a small measurable effect on blood sugar levels) will actually worsen their diabetes. Additionally, it will cause diabetes to develop in those individuals who are suffering from insulin resistance from chronic, excess daily ingestion of fructose.

The medical myth of fructose is that while we may think that it is a good, natural thing to ingest several servings of fresh fruit and their products (such as fruit smoothies, fruit juice and the like) every day, that very consumption is actually creating or adding to the problem of insulin resistance, obesity with its numerous associated diseases, and type II diabetes. While it may seem healthy to eat these foods as they are a good source of vitamins and minerals, they actually cause our health to decline if we follow the present U.S. Department of Agriculture recommendations. Not only do we need to dramatically reduce our consumption of table sugar and high fructose corn syrup, we also need to keep our intake of fructose from fruit sources in check as well. **Our**

total daily intake of fructose derived from all sources needs to be limited to 12-18 grams (12-15 per woman, 15-8 per man) or less per day. The glycemic index does not help us with fructose. This index was developed solely for the management of blood sugar levels in diabetics. Education about fructose and the consequences of excess, daily consumption is the key to helping us achieve a healthier state of being.

Pearls

- Fructose has a low glycemic index, yet it is the primary cause of insulin resistance and type II diabetes when consumed in chronic excess.

- The glycemic index was developed to help diabetics manage their diabetes. Fructose creates a paradox for diabetics as it causes and worsens the disease.

"There is nothing as mysterious as something clearly seen." *Robert Frost*

Chapter 16

Understanding the Food Label

J ust as it can be a daunting task to sort out medical myths from facts, understanding the labeling of ingredients in foods that you consume on a daily basis can be very challenging. Additionally, you often need a magnifying glass to even see the microscopically printed labels. The purpose of this chapter is to take apart the food labels found on commercially prepared foods line by line, so that you will become a more educated consumer as it relates to your nutrition. This is very important when you are trying to figure out how much fructose is present in a specific food product. If a large quantity of fructose is present, you may want to look for an alternative product that contains much lower quantities of this sugar. As an example, I went to the store the other day and picked up cocktail sauce for fresh shrimp. The first bottle of sauce I grabbed off the grocery shelf had 28 grams of sugar carbohydrates per serving. Wow, one serving and I would blow my entire day's allotment of sugar carbs with cocktail sauce. I looked through the other four brands on the shelf. One brand had a mere four grams of sugar per serving. This seemed much more reasonable, so I purchased that brand.

At this juncture, go to your cupboard or pantry and pull out some sort of processed food box, can or carton and refer to it as you read this chapter. I can promise you that if you do this you will come away with a much better understanding about food labeling and its pitfalls of interpretation.

There are two major parts to the food label. The first is the **"nutrition facts"** section and the other is the **"ingredients"** list. It is imperative to look at both parts to understand what you are actually purchasing. I will give you specific examples as we progress through the label. It is important at the outset to understand that the food labels are not all-inclusive for all the vitamins, minerals, water content, types of specific sugars or types of essential fatty acids present. Often, the label is quite misleading.

Let us look at the "nutrition facts" label. The first thing to notice when you pick up a package, carton, bottle or can of a food is how many servings and the size of the serving noted just under the "nutrition facts" label. Why is this important? Because you may look at a large box of crackers (containing hundreds of those tasty morsels) only to realize that two-to-five crackers is a "serving size." Perhaps for a bird! That is very important when you grab a handful of the crackers, as you may have several "servings" in that paw, let alone after the third handful. Be careful because you could easily consume hundreds, if not thousands of extra calories per day without even realizing it, just because of easy access to a large quantity of a loosely packaged food product.

Probably the most important line of the food label is the next one below the serving size. It is a very small line that says **"amount per serving."** This is a deadly term because it is the line that allows the food industry to mislead us with the blessings of the federal government. At this point you have to become a walking calculator as the food label does not tell you how many calories or how much of a substance is actually in the container (unless the container only contains one serving). I am looking at a can of french fried onions like the ones you put on top of green bean casserole. The serving size is two tablespoons (who knows if that is a level tablespoon, a packed tablespoon, a fluffy tablespoon as the onions fluff up, etc.) and there are 11 servings per container. So if I "realistically" eat three tablespoons of the onions on my helping of casserole, I am consuming one and a half servings. I now have to figure out the contents of a serving and multiply it by one and a half to figure out the calories, carbs, grams of fat, etc., for my "realistic" serving.

In today's supermarket very few packages contain only one serving. If you look at a can of soup, it will typically fill one soup bowl and yet it says on the label that it is two servings. You have just consumed twice the amount of everything listed on the nutrition facts portion of the label. Likewise, five Ritz crackers is a single serving. If you are like me you could easily consume a dozen or more in one sitting while eating your salami and cheese. Now you have to multiply the ingredients of the label by the number of crackers consumed, divided by five crackers per serving, and on and on and on. Instead, you just eat the crackers, salami and cheese and don't really try to figure it all out.

The next line after the "amount per serving" is the "calories and calories from fat" line. Again, remember that this is "calories and calories from fat" per serving, not per container (unless the container only contains one serving). You now have to quickly look back up to the servings per container line to see how many calories and fat calories you will realistically consume if you polish off the whole can of soup, bag of chips, etc. You have to multiply the number of servings by the total calories to know how many calories are in the container. One additional thought: I know of no one who counts crackers or cookies when they are actually devouring them unless they are actively dieting. They just consume a handful or three.

Below the calories line is a "total fat" grouping broken down into saturated fat and trans fat. Again, this is always referring back up to "amount per serving." The total fat routinely does not total up to the saturated fat and trans fat amounts listed below, because there are other types of fat that they do not define in the food label for you. Interestingly there are two essential fats needed to maintain human health. These are omega-3 and omega-6 fatty acids. These two fats need to be present in your diet in a two-to-one ratio in order to maintain proper health (see my first book). Yet, the content of these two essential fats is not even listed on the label.

One of the most misleading aspects of the nutrition facts of the food label is that it has allowed food manufacturers to deceive you as it relates to the trans fat label. The food label may claim zero grams of trans fat per serving so long as the amount of trans fat per serving is less than 500 mg. Why is it so critical for you to understand this fact? Several reasons. **First**, rarely does anyone ever consume only one serving size. Because of this you are consuming a significant amount of trans fats even if it is fewer than 500 mg per serving. **Second**, manufactured trans fats cause heart disease and several types of cancers and are associated with several other types of inflammatory diseases that affect the body. **Third**, some foods have only manufactured trans fats as their source of fat. An example of this is Ritz crackers or animal crackers. The label on these food items clearly states "zero grams trans fats," yet the fat listed in the ingredients section is partially hydrogenated vegetable oil. This is a manufactured trans fat. I just use these as examples, but the grocery store is full of many others. A container of Crisco shortening is the original trans fat. I recently read the label on a can of the shortening and it said zero grams trans fat per serving.

Another misleading aspect of trans fat labeling as it relates to the food label is that there is no distinction between natural trans fats versus manufactured trans fats. Cattle are what are known as ruminants. Ruminants consume their food and then rechew the food over the next several hours by regurgitating the food, grinding it and mixing it with their saliva and other gastric contents. If the cow consumes grass as its primary food, its intestinal bacteria are mixed with the grass during the rumination process.

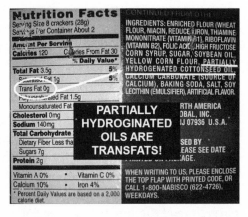

The bacteria initiate fermentation of the grass, and natural Trans fats are generated by this method of digestion. These natural trans fats (also called conjugated linoleic acid or CLAs) are then incorporated into the meat and milk of the cow. These natural trans fats are actually beneficial to human physiology. Studies reveal that natural trans fats reduce the risk of developing heart disease, obesity and cancer. Yet, if the diet of the cow is changed from grass to corn silage the natural trans fats disappear. The intestinal bacteria no longer produce the natural trans fats.

If you read a food label of a ground sirloin burger from a grocery store, you may immediately note that each patty contains up to 1.5 grams of trans fat per serving. Most of us

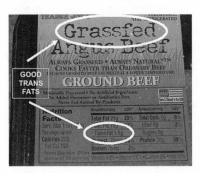

do not understand that trans fat found in meat from cattle only contains natural trans fats (CLAs). You might think that this beef patty is unhealthy when in fact it actually contains a type of fat that reduces your risk of developing heart disease, obesity and cancer.

So, you go back to your salami, cheese and crackers (the ones with zero grams trans fat per serving that is actually giving you several grams of manufactured trans fats in the end) instead of eating the burger from a grass fed beef cow that would be quite beneficial to your health. The take-home message here is that if the food label on the meat tells you that trans fats are present, these natural trans fats are good for you, while food labels that contain manufactured trans fats do not even have to tell you if they are present unless they have quantities that exceed 500 mg per serving. Either manipulate the serving size or keep the manufactured trans fat just under 500 mg per serving (say 498 mg) and you will never know the truth, unless you get out your magnifying glass to read the ingredients portion of the food label. (This is where they tell you what kind of fat has been added to the food product.) But, I will come back to this more in a moment.

The next line is the amount of cholesterol per serving. Another medical myth is the importance of this fat. Studies show that an individual can eat a diet that consists of only chicken eggs (a high cholesterol diet) and that individual will have a normal blood cholesterol level. Likewise, as noted previously, similar investigations of the Masai and Sumbaro Indians of Africa and Greenland Eskimos all show normal serum cholesterols. These three groups of people live on a very high fat, high cholesterol diet, yet they have minimal heart disease and normal serum cholesterol levels. It is only when they adopt the westernized high carbohydrate, high trans fat diet that their serum cholesterol levels rise, and their risk of heart disease worsens.

A Swedish cardiologist reviewed every major research paper ever published concerning the myths surrounding cholesterol. See the bibliography if you want to learn more specific details, but suffice it to say, medical science now knows that the bad LDL cholesterol levels rise with the ingestion of manufactured trans fats and chronic, excess fructose consumption. The food label does not educate us about the first of these, and it does not tell us how much fructose is present in the food product we are about to consume. Whether a food stuff contains cholesterol is not really important as it is broken down by our intestine into basic building blocks of metabolism and is never absorbed as cholesterol. The liver synthesizes the necessary cholesterol when our bodies require it to do so. Unfortunately, it also produces bad LDL cholesterol when we eat the wrong foods as mentioned above. Bad LDL cholesterol levels are only indicative of a metabolism gone awry, not that you are consuming cholesterol in your diet.

After the cholesterol entry, we see how much sodium is present in a serving. As you learned earlier in the book, if you have consumed enough fructose to turn on the metabolic syndrome, your kidneys will cause you to hold on to sodium (salt) which then leads to water retention. This will lead to high blood pressure. Sodium is an issue only if you have underlying metabolic syndrome, kidney disease (probably caused by the metabolic syndrome) or advanced heart or liver disease. The big push by the Food and Drug Administration at the time of this book is to decrease the amount of sodium (salt) served in restaurants. Various levels of government want to drastically reduce sodium content of processed food as well. Forget the cause of the sodium problem; just bandage the effect of chronic, excess fructose ingestion is what they seem to be saying. This all seems a bit backward to me.

I must say that I am not against reducing the salt content in many processed foods as they often contain excessive amounts of sodium. It is just that reducing salt in the Western diet is not stopping the problem of excess fructose-stimulated uric acid production that leads to salt retention.

The next section of the nutrition facts label is quite relevant to this book. It is the "total carbohydrate" information, which is further broken down into fiber and sugars. This is another very difficult section to understand unless you are informed about carbohydrates. Let me explain.

The fiber portion is fairly easy. This is the portion of the total carbohydrates that comes from plant fiber such as celluloses, gums or brans. While the label does not tell you the type of fiber present, the ingredient list may give you some clues. The list may actually name a specific fiber such as guar gum, oat bran, etc. Different fibers cause various intestinal reactions such as bloating, stool formation, gas formation and the like. Additionally, some fibers cause almost no intestinal complaints in one person and significant symptoms in another.

The sugar carbohydrates are more difficult to define and understand. You have to know what the ingredients are, and which ingredients are sugar carbohydrates or contain sugar carbohydrates. Further, you then must estimate the approximate content of the various sugar carbohydrates in the food product. You see, according to the food label, sugar carbohydrates encompass table sugar (sucrose), high fructose corn syrup, starches, milk sugar (lactose), malted sugar, fructose, glucose, galactose, sugar alcohols, fruit juice sugars, fruit puree and everything in between. It does not tell you how much of any of these specific sugar carbohydrates is present. If you understand that table sugar is 50% fructose, you can deduce that 50% of the sugar carbohydrates are fructose if table sugar is the only sugar carbohydrate in the ingredient list. Unfortunately, many food products contain several sources of sugar carbohydrates, and the food label does not share which ingredient contains which sugar carbohydrate or how much of a given sugar carbohydrate is present. As you now know from reading this book, it matters to you if you are trying to limit your fructose intake.

Let me shed more light on this issue by providing you with some examples that deal with the confusion that surrounds sugar carbohydrates. If you look at the food label on a dairy product, such as most cheeses, fruit-free yogurt, cottage cheese or milk you will often see sugar carbohydrates varying from zero to 15 grams per serving (depending on the producer). Yet, all of these sugar carbohydrates found in most of these products are glucose, galactose or lactose (milk sugar). There is no fructose present in any of these dairy products (other than a small amount of fructose in a few cheeses). The sugar carbohydrates present in unsweetened dairy items do not cause the metabolic syndrome. At the same time, fruit-sweetened yogurt may contain up to 25 grams of sugar carbohydrate per serving. The problem is that the food label does not have to inform you about the fructose content versus the glucose and galactose content in that container of yogurt. Because of this, you are left guessing about how much fructose is present, even though the ingredients will list fruit, fruit juice and the like that has been added to the yogurt.

Another very confusing section of the grocery store to decipher the sugar carbohydrate content in foods is the bakery. You see, starches found in flour account for the total and the sugar carbohydrates. They contain total carbohydrates comprised of fiber carbohydrates (bran, etc.) and sugar carbohydrates (the starch). Additionally, you must read through the ingredients to see if the bread was sweetened with table sugar (cane sugar, sucrose, etc.), high fructose corn syrup, fruit juice, honey or raisin puree and the like. These sugar carbohydrates are added to the starch component of the flour to make up the sugar carbohydrate quantity listed.

You are left with the task of trying to separate out the amount of sugar carbohydrates in each of these ingredients from the starch and fiber, before you can try to figure out how much of the sugar is actually fructose. This is not possible based on the information provided to you on the food label. Once you have an estimate of the fructose content, you still have to remember the distinction between a serving size and what you are going to eat. How often do you eat a sandwich made from a single slice (one serving) of bread? Finally, you may then be able to make the estimate of the fructose content for your portion size. Is it any wonder why we consume so much fructose without even realizing that we are doing so? Nobody is going to go through all the gyrations to try to figure out how much fructose they are consuming. It would be much more informative to the consumer if the food label just listed the fructose content. My approach, now that I have modified my diet to a low fructose menu, is to forego consuming many of these food products altogether as there are alternative foods that taste just as good.

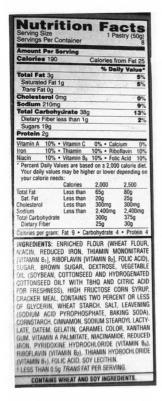

As can be seen from this food label, there are 19 grams of sugar included in a single serving as described in the nutrition facts. Five ingredients: flour (contains starch), sugar, brown sugar, dextrose, and high fructose corn syrup all contain sugars. The food label does not allow you to determine how much fructose is present in the serving. You are left to guess. My suggestion is to estimate the fructose content by cutting the number in half; sugar, brown sugar and high fructose corn syrup contain about 50% fructose. This means that a serving has about 10 grams of fructose. While this overestimates the fructose content, especially with dairy products, you can adjust your calculations as you learn the fructose contents of more and more foods.

The next part of the food label defines the quantity of protein present. There is no further definition as to the source of the protein. To figure this out you must again return to your magnifying glass and look through the ingredient list to try to figure out which ones contain the protein. You may see ingredients such as milk whey, soy protein, egg white solids and the list goes on ad infinitum. Good luck figuring all that, especially if you have a specific food allergy or dietary need.

The next to the last part of the nutrition facts section informs you of the vitamin A, vitamin C, calcium and iron content per serving. As you learned from the nutrition chapter there are several other essential vitamins and minerals, but the label tells you nothing of their contents. I could argue that there are several others very important for adequate nutrition, but I won't. I just advise my patients to take a good quality multivitamin daily so that they won't be deficient in any of them.

Well, if this hasn't been confusing enough, the final portion of the nutrition section is a small print labeling that says that all of the above information of the percent daily value of the food is based on a 2000 calorie diet. Good luck trying to convert all the percentages if you consume 850 calories one day, 3200 calories another, and 1500 calories the next. As you can see, you are presented with another daunting task.

Finally, I want to talk about the magnifying glass section (the ingredient list) for just a bit more. As you can see, you cannot truly analyze the nutrition facts section without knowing the ingredients as both lists are intricately tied to each other. You need to look at the ingredients to see how it impacts the components on the nutrition list. Also, many of the ingredients are items that are not in our cultural vocabulary. Let me list a few: hydrolyzed yeast extract, disodium inosinate, guar gum, xanthum gum, TBHQ, monosodium glutamate, silicon dioxide, whey, hydrolyzed corn gluten, sodium tripolyphosphate, hydrolyzed soy protein. The list could go on for pages. I would argue that most people do not know what most of the ingredients in a food product are, let alone whether they contain fat, protein or carbohydrates.

You can see how overwhelming it is to try interpreting the food label, let alone attempting to figure out how much fructose is present in the product you are about to consume. In a later chapter I will give you some encouraging advice about a reasonable approach to this daunting task.

Pearls

- The food label is a complicated and often misleading information marker found on all processed foods.
- It is imperative that you learn how to interpret this label in order to avoid consuming trans fats and excess fructose.

"There is no substitute for accurate knowledge."
Lee Iacocca

Chapter 17

How Sweet It Is: Artificial Sweeteners

Nearly every day in my gastroenterology clinic a patient asks me what they can use as a substitute for high fructose corn syrup, sugar or other fructose-containing products when they are trying to reduce their fructose intake, but still want to nurture their sweet taste buds. Because of those constant inquiries, I thought I should include a short chapter on the various artificial sweeteners presently on the market. While I cannot provide a complete expose' on every aspect of this topic, here is a broad overview to enhance your understanding of the products presently available in the supermarket.

All artificial sweeteners are regulated by the U.S. Food and Drug Administration (FDA). These sweeteners are approved by the FDA as a sugar substitute to sweeten foods and beverages. There are presently six such sweeteners (also referred to as high intensity sweeteners) approved by the FDA for human consumption. They include: acesulfame potassium, aspartame, neotame, saccharin, stevia, and sucralose. Technically stevia is not an artificial sweetener as it is a sweetener that is extracted from the leaves of the stevia plant. Each of these high intensity sweeteners is much sweeter than table sugar so much smaller quantities can be used to sweeten food products. Many other artificial sweeteners are used in other nations and some are under review by the FDA for possible release into the U.S. commodity market in the future.

The artificial sweetener market is fierce, and this leads to a major challenge when you attempt to determine their long term safety with prolonged human consumption. There is a continual barrage of "bad press" appearing on the Internet concerning any of these products. While I am not an expert on any of these products, I have read numerous articles over the years in an attempt to stay abreast of the safety issues that surround artificial sweeteners. One thing for certain is that they are not going to disappear from the supermarket because of the demand for a calorie-free sweetener in a population with an ever growing waistline.

Artificial sweeteners are not new to the marketplace. The first of these sweeteners was discovered in 1879. A researcher in Baltimore, Maryland, accidently spilled a chemical derivative of coal tar on his hand. He licked it off and noted that it was sweet. Further investigation led to the discovery of saccharin. Since that time there has been a steady stream of new products developed the world over all attempting to become the perfect sugar substitute. Table 1 gives you the sweetener, its brand name, and its sweetness compared to sugar.

Some of the benefits of consuming artificial sweeteners include: no calories added to the food or beverage for many of the high intensity sweeteners; no dental cavities with regular consumption contrary to fructose-containing sugars; less cost to the manufacturer as they are much less expensive than sugar; and minimal effect on blood sugar in diabetics. It is important to note that the "sugar-free" label does not mean calorie free. An example is that sucralose contains between two and three calories per packet compared with 12 calories per packet for table sugar. However, sucralose does not

Table 1. Comparison of Sweeteners to Sugar

Sweetener	Brand Name	Relative Sweetness to Sugar
Acesulfame	Sunett, Sweet One	200 X
Acesulfame	Sunett, Sweet One	200 X
Aspartame	Nutrasweet, Equal	200 X
Neotame	None Yet	7000-13,000 X
Saccharine	Sweet'N Low, Sweet Twin	200-700 X
Stevia	Truvia, Trusweet, PureVia	300 X
Sucralose	Splenda, Apriva	600 X

induce the metabolic syndrome or raise your serum uric acid with regular intake like fructose-containing sugars.

The flip side is that there are constant allegations in the press about various side effects, toxicities, and the cause of various cancers, mutations and hormonal problems related to the various sweeteners. When you muddle through many of the allegations, they are often derived from some animal or Petri dish study where amazingly high concentrations of the artificial sweetener are injected into animal bladders (and the like) and then the animal develops a bladder cancer. The FDA has been aggressively monitoring the safety of these products for most of the 20th and now the 21st century, and all of them remain on the market.

The only label warning found on any of these artificial sweeteners is the one found on aspartame. This is because of the possibility of an adverse reaction in patients who suffer from a rare inherited disorder called phenylketonuria. These individuals cannot metabolize aspartame and it can become toxic for them.

There is no magic to any one artificial sweetener. I have heard of many complaints by individuals concerning virtually all of these sweeteners, so you just have to give the various ones a try to see if there is one tolerable for you. If one bothers you, try another. To date, there is no scientific evidence to warrant removing any of them from the market. The FDA as well as the food industry have performed and reviewed hundreds of toxicology and clinical projects. Additionally, they have been reviewing massive amounts of after-marketing data for decades and it has not led to the removal of artificial sweeteners from the supermarket. Many other nations are also constantly monitoring the artificial sweetener market for problems.

While I do not advocate for any one artificial sweetener, I would strongly encourage their use over chronic, excess fructose intake. I know the outcome of the latter, and to date, there is no data to raise significant health concerns in spite of decades of use, especially when compared to foods and beverages filled with sugars full of fructose.

Pearls

- Artificial sweeteners do not cause the metabolic syndrome.

- While these sweeteners may cause side effects in an individual, they are far safer than the effects of chronic, excess fructose ingestion.

"If you are planning for a year, sow rice;
if you are planning for a decade, plant trees;
if you are planning for a lifetime, educate people."
Chinese proverb

Chapter 18

Dieting Versus
Reduced Fructose Living

One of my nurses is trim and fit. She exercises regularly; she is very conscientious about her diet; she is moderate in nearly every aspect of her daily living. Yet, she has mild high blood pressure, her bad LDL cholesterol is elevated, and she is developing insulin resistance. She is frustrated because she takes such good care of herself. I discussed her diet with her. She is nearly a vegetarian, but she begins each day with a large, homemade fruit smoothie chock full of various berries, fruits, and other nutritious ingredients. The problem is that her smoothie contains around 50 grams of fructose, not from high fructose corn syrup, honey or sugar; rather, from the fruits and berries. Her liver can process only 12-15 grams per day (15-18 grams per day for a male) without turning on the metabolic syndrome.

I want to share one more experience I had with my sister. We had been discussing the background information about this book, and she was very enthusiastic in applying its concepts to her diet. She was interested in shedding a few pounds after the holidays from enjoying Christmas cookies, candies and the like. She became a bit frustrated when she did not rapidly lose weight by going through a fructose fast.

We had another discussion about the distinction between weight loss and fructose reduction. Reducing fructose after a fructose fast reverses the metabolic syndrome enzymes in the liver. After this is accomplished, maintaining a reduction of fructose to levels that do not turn them back on prevents conversion of fructose to body fat. But, to lose weight, we need to do several things.

First, we need to determine how many total calories we are consuming daily. If our caloric intake is 3000 calories per day and our body is only burning up 1500 calories, we will gain weight. It doesn't matter whether we have eliminated all the fructose from our diet. Once we have established a realistic caloric need for our body, we need to reduce our daily intake of food to a bit lower than our body's needs; otherwise we will only maintain weight.

Second, we need to increase our metabolic activity. This stimulation in our metabolism causes our body to burn off those calories we are consuming in a more efficient way. In turn, we will begin to lose weight faster than if we had only reduced the total calorie intake. How do we increase our metabolic rate? We can eat certain foods that take a lot of energy when they are consumed. A few examples are drinking iced beverages rather than room temperature beverages. The body must warm that beverage to body temperature. That requires increased metabolism expenses. Foods such as broccoli, cauliflower and brussel sprouts require a significant amount of metabolic energy to extract the nutrition from them. Finally, increased physical activity stimulates our metabolic rate. We need about 20-30 minutes of aerobic activity daily in order to achieve this increase. This would include brisk walking, jogging, bicycling, step aerobics, hot yoga, dancing, swimming, gardening, etc. Numerous aerobic programs have been developed to meet just about anybody's interests, abilities, and time constraints. The most important things to remember with aerobic exercise are that you need to increase your heart rate to the point that your body warms up (unless cooled by the swimming pool, outdoor air, etc.) and that it is performed at least five days per week. Studies show that both of these principles are important for weight loss from aerobic activity.

Third, the human body requires use to remain healthy. If you do not keep your muscles strong, they atrophy, and your strength decreases. Building muscle strength increases your overall health, but it also increases your metabolic activity. Fascinating studies show that it takes only three consecutive days of bed rest to cause your body's strength to plummet. Additionally, your body can build muscle strength and mass even into your nineties with appropriate exercise.

Finally, you need to consume all the essential nutrients daily that your body can lose weight while you remain in good health. You can starve yourself of calories in an attempt to lose weight, but you could suffer nerve, brain or muscle damage during your weight loss if not done properly. I would refer you back to the nutrition chapter for the specifics; however, you need a vitamin with minerals, plenty of fluids, enough protein and essential fatty acids to maintain your health while you are dieting.

If you have an increased amount of body fat even though you have eliminated fructose excess from your diet, this is not healthy. Numerous diseases are strongly associated with obesity as listed in table 1 below.

Table 1. Diseases Associated with Obesity

Cancers	Breast Colon Esophagus Gallbladder	Liver Pancreas Prostate Uterus
Cardiovascular	Heart Disease High Blood Pressure Congestive Heart Failure Deep Vein Thrombosis (blood clots in the leg veins) Pulmonary Embolism (blood clots in the lungs) Varicose Veins	
Dermatologic	Increased Pigmentation of the Skin Facial Hair Skin Infections Stretch Marks Poor Circulation	
Digestive	Esophageal Reflux Barrett's Esophagus (precancerous change of esophagus) Gallstones Pancreatitis Colon Polyps (precancerous growths in the colon) Fatty Liver Cirrhosis Liver Failure	

Endocrine	Type II Diabetes/Insulin Resistance Metabolic Syndrome Sexual Impotence Polycystic Ovary Syndrome Vitamin D Deficiency Menstrual Irregularity Infertility Elevated Uric Acid/Gout
Genitourinary	Urinary Incontinence Kidney Damage/Kidney Failure Kidney Stones
Musculoskeletal	Low Back Pain Loss of Mobility Gouty Arthritis Degenerative Arthritis
Neurologic	Dementia Strokes
Psychologic	Depression Eating Disorders (bulimia, anorexia nervosa, etc.)
Pulmonary	Pulmonary Hypertension (lung high blood pressure) Asthma Obstructive Sleep Apnea Right Heart Failure

As you can see, the body does not do well with obesity. Obesity-related diseases are now the leading cause of death on the planet. The obesity incidence doubled in America between 1980 and 2005. Additionally, those who are considered overweight increased 300%. Approximately 365,000 preventable deaths were attributed to obesity in 2000, and the numbers of all these conditions continues to rise. While many factors contribute to obesity, chronic, excess fructose consumption is a major player.

At the same time that people that are obese suffer from many ailments, they also spend more time and money on healthcare. A report in 2009 revealed that obese individuals spend 42% more on healthcare than non-obese people. That year it accounted for $1400 more for obese individuals. Obesity-related healthcare costs account for tens of billions of dollars annually, and this number is increasing each year. The individual (like I mentioned at the outset of this chapter) who is not obese, but is suffering from the metabolic effects of chronic, excess fructose ingestion can also have medical costs that are staggering and frustrating.

Obesity is defined in various ways, but the current medical standard is the body mass index (BMI). The body mass index is defined as your weight in kilograms divided by your height in meters squared. This is not very user friendly as most of us don't use kilograms or meters in our daily affairs. For those of us who are comfortable with pounds, inches and feet, the formula can be modified to our understanding. You multiply your weight in pounds by 703 and divide by your height in inches squared; alternatively, multiple your weight in pounds by 4.88 and divide this by your height in feet squared. (Even this seems awkward so I have included the following table for your reference.)

Table 2. Body Mass Index

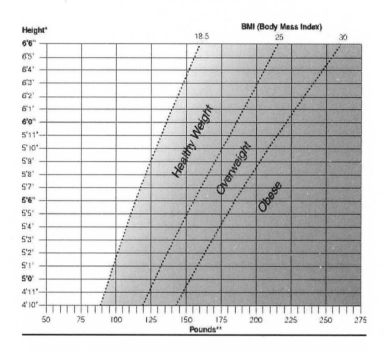

Obesity is defined as a BMI of 30 or higher. Individuals who are muscular or pregnant do not fit into the BMI measurement scheme very well. For the pregnant individual, this is a transient state that should not govern long-term weight management. For the muscular individual, one would have to look to other measurement schemes to determine whether they are obese. The accuracy of the BMI for individuals in the intermediate overweight range (BMI 25-29.59), in men and in the elderly does not have very good applicability for heart disease and its associated death risks. In fact, a review of 40 published studies showed that individuals with a normal BMI were at higher risk of heart disease than these other groups. It is clear from the findings from this many studies that there are other issues than just obesity that must be con-

181

sidered as risk factors for specific diseases. For example, you do not have to be obese just because you eat excess fructose or manufactured trans fats. Yet, we know that consuming too much of these substances will dramatically increase your risk of heart disease independent of obesity.

If you are trying to reduce fructose intake but do not have a weight problem, you are fortunate. All you need to do is turn off the metabolic enzymes in the liver, then return to healthy living. But, if you are like two-thirds of the American population that needs to shed pounds, then you need to reduce fructose intake and lose weight. This latter issue is outlined earlier in the chapter. The next chapter will focus on the former in more detail.

Pearls

- Obesity due to the metabolic syndrome is associated with many chronic diseases.

- Decreasing fructose alone may not be adequate to reduce your weight if you are obese and are suffering from the metabolic syndrome.

- In addition to decreased fructose intake, reduction in total caloric intake, increasing our metabolic activity through aerobic exercise, increasing muscle mass by strengthening workouts and consuming all your essential nutrients are necessary to achieve sustained weight loss.

"The way to get started is to quit talking and begin doing." *Walt Disney*

Chapter 19

Initiating the Reduced Fructose Lifestyle

T wo-thirds of the American population is suffering from various aspects of the metabolic syndrome because of chronic, excess fructose ingestion. Additionally, an even higher percentage is overweight or obese according to recent surveys. As you examine your own health, you first need to determine if you suffer from the former or both of these problems. First, determine your weight loss needs by looking up your body mass index from the table in the previous chapter. If you do not need to lose weight but are suffering from high blood pressure, elevated blood triglycerides, abnormal blood levels of good (HDL) and bad (LDL) cholesterol, elevated blood uric acid levels, or borderline diabetes, then your metabolic syndrome enzymes have been activated because of chronic, excess fructose ingestion. They need to be inactivated.

The number one goal in initiating a reduced fructose lifestyle is to turn off the liver enzymes that are creating metabolic chaos. This requires a complete elimination of all fructose from your diet for a three week period. If you just reduce fructose intake the liver enzymes may continue to function. It is analogous to a dripping faucet. If the water spigot is turned down but water is still coming out, then the water is not turned off. The same concept must be applied to turning off the metabolic syndrome pathways.

In order for you to turn off the faucet you need to **eliminate** all of the following food items for a period long enough to ensure liver enzyme shutdown:

All Fruits
All Fruit Juices
All Vegetables
All Breads except for Sour Dough and French Breads
All Honey
All Sugar
All High Fructose Corn Syrup
All Cookies, Candies, Cakes, Ice Cream
All Foods that Contain Sugar Carbohydrates on the Nutrition Label
All Sugar- or High Fructose Corn Syrup-Sweetened Beverages

If there is any doubt whether you can eat it, you should not consume it because any fructose during this three week fructose fast will keep the liver enzymes activated. An example of this is alcohol. Many alcoholic beverages have been sugar fortified. Cocktail drinks are routinely sweetened with fructose-containing sugars. Fortified wines such as Port and Madeira, as well as many types of champagne, contain fructose. Additionally, beer leads to uric acid production independent of fructose metabolism. Because of complicated metabolic issues surrounding alcohol, it is better to eliminate these libations for the three week period rather than chance the failure of turning off the dripping faucet.

What can you eat during this period? Here is a list of fructose-free foods that can be consumed:

All Meats (poultry, fish, beef, pork, etc.)
Sugar-Free Pastas
Sugar-Free Sour Dough Bread
Sugar-Free French Bread
Dairy Products (except sweetened yogurt, some cheese)
Eggs
Beverages Sweetened with Artificial Sweeteners

As you can see, this is a rather limited diet for the three weeks while you are fasting from all fructose. If there is any question concerning the fructose content of something you want to include in your diet, refer back to the fructose tables in Chapter 9.

Because many of the foods and beverages that contain fructose also contain many essential vitamins and minerals, you will need to supplement your diet with a good quality multivitamin daily. Additionally, our diet is deficient in omega-3 fatty acids. You will want to add an omega-3 fatty acid supplement (fish oil or flax seed oil) with each meal. Two to three capsules at the beginning of each meal is typically adequate to meet your body's needs. If you are eating fish for your entree you can forego supplementation for that meal.

Remember also that you will feel the effects of fasting from fructose for a few days. Your brain has become addicted to fructose, and there will be a withdrawal period that may cause you to have various symptoms, such as light headedness, continued hunger even with adequate calorie intake, craving for anything sweet, etc. Your resolve will be challenged for those few days to stick with the fructose fast. But, it will be worth it to turn off the liver enzymes that lead to the metabolic syndrome.

While you are going through the fructose fast, you also need to drink plenty of water, and always avoid all trans fats (hydrogenated or partially hydrogenated oils).

Once you have made it through the three weeks of misery from no fruits, juices and sweets of all sorts, you can now add vegetables back into your diet. But, contrary to the advice of the federal government, **do not resume consuming several servings of fruit or fruit juice per day.** Additionally, do not return to consuming all of the sweets of your past diet. If you do, you will turn the liver enzymes back on and you will have to start over.

To Recap:
(1) **Avoid All Fructose** for Three Weeks
(2) **Take a Multivitamin** Daily
(3) **Take an Omega-3 Fatty Acid Supplement** with each Meal
(4) **Drink Plenty of Fluids**
(5) **Avoid All trans Fats** (hydrogenated or partially hydrogenated vegetable oils)
(6) **Resume Fructose in a Reduced Amount** of less than 12-18 Grams per Day after Three Weeks (12-15 per female, 15-18 per male)

Now what you need to do is develop an understanding of how much fructose is present in many of the foods you routinely eat. You need to set up a fructose budget so that you consume 12-18 grams of fructose per day (12-15 grams per female, 15-18 grams per male). This is where you need to return to the chapter that defines the amount of fructose found in commonly consumed foods. It is essential that you learn the fructose contents of your favorites. Then, learn to limit your daily consumption of fructose so that you do not reactivate the liver enzymes responsible for the metabolic syndrome.

Let us now return to the issue of weight loss. If you also need to lose a few pounds, you will need to count total calories as well as fructose carbohydrates. An important way to initiate weight loss along with shutting down fructose metabolism is to be judicious after the three week fast when you start consuming fructose carbohydrates again. One of the best ways of doing this is to add vegetables without adding fruits or fruit juices. As I pointed out earlier, consuming many vegetables increases your metabolic rate. An increased metabolic rate stimulates weight loss if you are consuming few enough total calories. Additionally, excess total carbohydrate intake leads directly to the production of fat if you are consuming more than you are burning off. There is a limited storage capacity of carbohydrates in the body in the form of glycogen. The liver and muscles are the two primary sites storing this excess blood sugar. Once all of the storage sites are full, the rest of the sugar is converted to fat.

Exercise burns up sugar. As the blood sugar starts to fall, the glycogen is mobilized and converted back to blood sugar to meet further energy needs. Once the glycogen storehouse has been depleted, your body can now start to burn off fat. The primary way to keep your glycogen levels low is to avoid carbohydrates high in starch (rice, potatoes, pastas, bread) and through exercise. In order to burn off built-up body fat, you need to participate in aerobic exercise. This is performed through physical exercise that increases the blood pressure, heart rate and body temperature without strenuously working muscles. Exercises such as brisk walking, jogging, cross-country skiing, bicycling, water aerobics, hot yoga and the like are good examples of aerobic exercise. Remember to participate in this type of exercise 5-6 times per week and work out to build up muscle strength 2-3 times per week.

Great snack foods that are low in fructose for active teens on the go include: nuts, vegetables, popcorn (not sweetened), baked potato chips, cheese sticks and unsweetened yogurt.

A final point that I would like to make is that it is easy for us to slip back to our previous ways of excess fructose intake. Because of this I would encourage you to go through a fructose fast after the Christmas holidays and again in the summer after the fresh fruit season. This way you can rest assured that you will remind yourself to continue with a **Reduced Fructose Lifestyle**.

Pearls

- Turning off the metabolic syndrome requires a three week fast from all fructose in your diet.
- Resume a reduced fructose diet indefinitely containing 12-18 grams per day (12-15 per female, 15-18 per male).

"An investment in knowledge pays the best dividend." *Benjamin Franklin*

Chapter 20

Let's Review

W e need to understand why the health of our nation has deteriorated so severely in the past twenty-five years. In order to do that we must first recognize the major changes in our diet; then we need to understand the contributions of those changes to the destruction of our health. This book (and my previous book concerning the changes in the fat composition of our diet) has attempted to educate you on both counts.

First, we have learned about the massive increase in excess daily ingestion of fructose. This increase has come through increased consumption of fruit, fruit juices and high fructose corn syrup. Fructose is a sugar that makes up a major portion of many fruits, 50% of table sugar and typically 55% of high fructose corn syrup found in many beverages at the supermarket. We have also dramatically increased the serving size of a given food or beverage over the past three decades. Part of this has been driven by the lack of appetite suppression that occurs with over consumption of fructose. We are then driven to eating larger portions in an attempt to feel full.

Fructose activates a series of enzymes in the liver that causes a metabolic change in the body. This change has been coined the metabolic syndrome. The metabolic syndrome leads to a series of disease processes that will shorten our life expectancy. These include: insulin resistance and type II diabetes, hypertension, elevated blood triglycerides, elevated bad (LDL) cholesterol, depressed good (HDL) cholesterol, heart disease, strokes, cancers, elevated blood uric acid levels, inflammatory arthritis and kidney failure. Additionally, it causes central obesity and numerous diseases associated with chronic, excess body weight.

As these metabolic changes occur from chronic excess fructose consumption, the health of many in the United States is suffering greatly. Now even children are feeling the ill effects of these metabolic changes. The sooner we recognize the metabolic syndrome transformation in our own body, the quicker we can make changes in our diet to reverse the metabolic processes. When we understand the long-term devastating effects that we are causing in our bodies, we can take steps to stop the damage, and reverse many of those effects.

Fructose fasting for three weeks is the key to turning off the liver enzymes that are causing the damage. While this can be a daunting task, we have strong motivation to accomplish this goal if we want to regain our health. The motivation may be weak if we do not understand the sources of fructose and the damage that will occur without making the necessary changes. As they say, with knowledge comes power, and with the knowledge contained in this (and my previous text) book you now have the power to take control of your own health in ways that could have medical benefits for you and future generations.

We have learned about the ubiquitous distribution of fructose in the Western diet. We have learned about the damage its chronic excess produces in our body, and we have learned how to turn it off. Most importantly, though is the maintenance of a reduced fructose lifestyle so that we do not revert back to the metabolic syndrome. It is a challenge but it is also a choice. And, the choice is yours and yours alone.

Hopefully, this book has enlightened you enough to help you make the right choice.

Good luck!

M. Frank Lyons II, M.D.

Bibliography

Ackerman, Z., et al. Fructose induced fatty liver disease: hepatic effects of blood pressure and plasma triglyceride reduction. Hypertension 2005; 45: 1012-18.

Akhavan, T., Anderson, G.H. Effects of glucose-to-fructose ratios in solutions on subjective satiety, food intake, and satiety hormones in young men. American Journal of Clinical Nutrition 2007; 86: 1354-63.

Ambrose, S.E. Undaunted Courage. Simon and Schuster, 1996.

Andersson, D.E., Nygren, A. Four cases of long-standing diarrhoea and colic pains cured by fructose-free diet—A pathogenic discussion. Acta Medica Scandinavia 1978; 203: 87-92.

Angelopoulos, T.J., Lowndes, J., Zukley, L., et al. The effect of high-fructose corn syrup consumption on triglycerides and uric Acid. Journal of Nutrition 2009; 139: 1242S-1245S.

Avena, N.M., Rada, P., Hoebel, B.G. Evidence for sugar addiction: behavioral and neurochemical effects of intermittent, excessive sugar intake. Neuroscience and Biobehavioral Reviews 2008; 32: 20-39.

Banks. W.A., et al. Triglycerides induce leptin resistance at the blood-brain barrier. Diabetes 2004; 53: 1253-60.

Bergreen, L. Over the Edge of the World: Magellan's Terrifying Circumnavigation of the Globe. HarperCollins, 2004.

Beyer, P.L., Caviar, E.M., McCallum, R.W. Fructose intake at current levels in the United States may cause gastrointestinal distress in normal adults. Journal of the American Dietetic Association 2005; 105:1559-66.

Bray, G.A. How bad is fructose? American Journal of Clinical Nutrition 2007; 86: 895-896.

Bray, G.A., Nielson, S.J., Popkin, B.M. Consumption of high fructose corn syrup in beverages may play a role in the epidemic of obesity. American Journal of Clinical Nutrition 2004; 79: 537-43.

Bray, G.A., Champagne, C.M. Beyond energy balance: There is more to obesity than kilocalories. Journal of the American Dietetic Association 2005; 105:S17-S23.

Brown, C.M., Dulloo, A.G., Montani, J.P. Sugary drinks in the pathogenesis of obesity and cardiovascular diseases. International Journal of Obesity 2008; 32:528-532.

Brown, C.M., Dulloo, A.G., Yepuri, G., et al. Fructose ingestion acutely elevates blood pressure in healthy young humans. American Journal of Physiology (Regulatory, Integrative, and comparative Physiology) 2008; 294: R730-R737.

Carmona, A., Freedland, R.A. Comparison among the lipogenic potential of various substrates in rat hepatocytes: the differential effects of fructose-containing diets on hepatic lipogenesis. The Journal of Nutrition 1989; 119: 1304-10.

Catenacci, V.A., Hill, J.O., Wyatt, H.R. The obesity epidemic. Clinics in Chest Medicine 2009; 30: 415-44.

Cha, S.H. Wolfgang, M., Tokutake, Y. et al. Differential effects of central fructose and glucose on hypothalamic malonyl-CoA and food intake. Proceedings of the National Academy of Science (USA) 2008; 105: 16871-75.

Chong, M.F. Mechanisms for the acute effect of fructose on postprandial lipemia. American Journal of Clinical Nutrition 2007; 85: 1511-20.

Choi H.K., Curhan, G. Soft Drinks, Fructose Consumption, and the Risk of Gout in Men: Prospective Cohort Study. British Medical Journal 2008; 336: 309-12.

Choi, J.W., Ford, E.S., Gao, X, et al. Sugar-Sweetened Soft Drinks, Diet Soft Drinks, and Serum Uric Acid Level: the Third National Health and Nutrition Examination Survey. Arthritis and Rheumatism 2008; 59: 109-16.

Cirillo, P., Gersch, M.S., Mu, W., et al. Ketohexokinase-dependent metabolism of fructose induces proinflammatory mediators in proximal tubular cells. Journal of the American Society of Nephrology 2009; 20: 545-53.

Cirillo, P., Sato, W., Reungjui, S., et al. Uric acid, the metabolic syndrome, and renal disease. Journal of the American Society of Nephrology 2006; 17: S165-S68.

Collison, K.S., et al. Diabetes of the liver: the link between nonalcoholic fatty liver disease and HFCS-55. Obesity 2009; 17: 657-662.

Dennison, B.A., Rockwell, H.L., Baker, S.L. Excess fruit juice consumption by preschool-aged children is associated with short stature and obesity. Pediatrics 1997: 99: 15-22.

Dessein, P.H., Shipton, E.A., Stanwix, A.E., et al. Beneficial effects of weight loss associated with moderate calorie/carbohydrate restriction, and increased proportional Iintake of protein and unsaturated fat on serum urate and lipoprotein levels in gout: A pilot study. Annals of Rheumatic Diseases 2000; 59: 539-43.

Dietz, W.H. Sugar-sweetened beverages, milk intake, and obesity in children and adolescents. Journal of Pediatrics 2006; 148: 152-54.

DiMeglio, D.P., Mattes, R.D. Liquid versus solid carbohydrate: effects on food Intake and body weight. International Journal of Obesity 2000; 24: 794-800.

Dirlewanger, M., Schneiter, P., Jequier, E. et al. Effects of fructose on hepatic glucose metabolism in humans. American Journal of Physiology, Endocrinology and Metabolism 200; 283: E545-E55.

Donnelly, R., Reed, M.J., Azhar, S., et al. Expression of the major isoenzyme of protein kinase-C in skeletal muscle, nPKC Theta, varies with muscle type and in response to fructose-induced insulin resistance. Endocrinology 1994; 135: 2369-74.

Elliott, S.S., Keim, N.L., Stern, J.S., et al. Fructose, weight gain, and the insulin resistance syndrome. American Journal of Clinical Nutrition 2002; 76: 911-22.

Faeh, D., et al. Effect of fructose overfeeding and fish oil administration on hepatic de novo lipogenesis and insulin sensitivity in healthy men. Diabetes 2005; 54: 1907-13.

Faith, M.S., Dennison, B.A., Edmunds, L.S., et al. Fruit juice intake predicts increased adiposity gain in children from low income families: weight status by environment interaction. Pediatrics 2006; 118: 2066-2075.

Feig, D.I. Sour notes on sweet drinks. Journal of Pediatrics 2009; 154: 783-84.

Feig, D.I., Johnson, R.J. Hyperuricemia in childhood primary hypertension. Hypertension 2003; 42: 247-52.

Feig, D.I., Kang, D., Johnson, R.J. Uric acid and cardiovascular risk. New England Journal of Medicine 2008; 359: 1811-21.

Feig, D.I., Soletsky, B., Johnson, R.J. Effect of allopurinol on blood pressure of adolescents with newly diagnosed essential hypertension: A randomized trial. Journal of the American Medical Association 2008; 300: 924-932.

Fernandez-Banares, F., Esteve-Pardo, M., de Leon, R., et al. Sugar malabsorption in functional bowel disease: Clinical Implications. American Journal of Gastroenterology 1993; 88: 2044-50.

Fox, I.H., Kelley, W.N. Studies on the mechanism of fructose-induced hyperuricemia in man. Metabolism 1972; 21: 713-21.

Foxx-Orenstein, A.E. Gastrointestinal symptoms and diseases related to obesity: An overview. Gastroenterology Clinics of North America 2010; 39: 23-37.

Fried, S.K., Rao, S.P. Sugars, hypertriglyceridemia, and cardiovascular disease. American Journal of Clinical Nutrition 2003; 78: 873S-80S.

Gaby, A.R., Adverse effects of dietary fructose. Alternative Medicine Reviews 2005; 10: 294-306.

Gao, X., Qi, L., Qiao, N., et al. Intake of added sugar and sugar-sweetened drink and serum uric acid concentration in U.S. men and women. Hypertension 2007; 50: 306-12.

Gersch, M.S., Mu, W., Cirillo, P., et al. Fructose, but not dextrose, accelerated the progression of chronic kidney disease. American Journal of Physiology. Renal Physiology 2007; 293: F1256-F61.

Goldberg, I.J. Hypertriglyceridemia: Impact and treatment. Endocrinology and Metabolism Clinics 2009; 38: 137-49.

Gross, L.S., Li, L., Ford, E.S., et al. Increased consumption of refined carbohydrates and the epidemic of type 2 diabetes in the United States: an ecologic assessment. American Journal of Clinical Nutrition 2004; 79: 774-79.

Hallfrisch, J. Metabolic effects of dietary fructose. The Federation of American Societies for Experimental Biology Journal 1990; 4: 2652-60.

Hallfrisch, J., Ellwood, K.C., Michaelis, S., et al. Effects of dietary fructose on plasma glucose and hormone responses in normal and hyperinsulinemic men. Journal of Nutrition 1983; 113: 1819-26.

Hamaguchi, M., Kojima, T., Takeda, N., et al. The Metabolic syndrome as a predictor of nonalcoholic fatty liver disease. Annals of Internal Medicine 2005:143: 722-28.

Havel, P.J. Dietary Fructose: Implications for dysregulation of energy homeostasis and lipid/carbohydrate metabolism. Nutrition Reviews 2005; 63:133-57.

Hwang, I.S., Ho, H., Hoffman, B.B., et al. Fructose-induced insulin resistance and hypertension in rats. Hypertension 1987; 10: 512-16.

Jacobson, M.F. High fructose corn syrup and the obesity epidemic. American Journal of Clinical Nutrition 2004; 80:1081.

Johnson, R.J., Perez-Pozo, S.E., Sautin, Y.Y., et al. Hypothesis: Could excessive fructose intake and uric acid cause type 2 diabetes? Endocrinology Reviews 2009; 30: 96-116.

Johnson, R.J., Segal, M.S., Sautin, Y., et al. Potential role of sugar (fructose) in the epidemic of hypertension, obesity and the metabolic syndrome, diabetes, kidney disease, and cardiovascular disease. American Journal Clinical Nutrition 2007; 86: 899-906.

Jurgens, H., Haass, W., Castaneda, T.R., et al. Consuming fructose-sweetened beverages increases body adiposity in mice. Obesity Research 2005; 13: 1146-56.

Kanarek, R.B., Orthen-Gambill, N. Differential effects of sucrose, fructose, and glucose on carbohydrate-induced obesity in rats. The Journal of Nutrition 1982; 112: 1546-54.

Kazumi, T., Vranic, M., Steiner, G. Triglyceride kinetics: Effects of dietary glucose, sucrose, or fructose alone or with hyperinsulinemia. American Journal of Physiology 1986; 250: E325-E30.

Keller, K.B., Lemberg, L. Obesity and the metabolic syndrome. American Journal of Critical Care. 2003; 12: 167-70.

Kelley, G.L., Allan, G., Azhar, S. High Dietary Fructose Induces a Hepatic Stress Response Resulting in Cholesterol and Lipid Dysregulation. Endocrinology 2004; 145: 548-55.

Koteish, A., Diehl, A.M. Animal models of steatosis. Seminars in Liver Disease 2001; 21: 89-104.

LA KA, Faeh, D., Stettler, R., et al. A 4-wk High fructose diet alters lipid metabolism without affecting insulin sensitivity or ectopic lipids in healthy humans. American Journal of Clinical Nutrition 2006; 84: 1374-79.

LA KA, Ith, M., Kreis R., et al. Fructose overconsumption causes dyslipidemia and ectopic lipid deposition in healthy subjects with and without a family history of type 2 diabetes. American Journal of Clinical Nutrition 2009; 89: 1760-65.

Le, K.A., Tappy, L. Metabolic effects of fructose. Current Opinion in Clinical Nutrition and Metabolic Care 2006; 9: 469-475.

Lim, J.S., Mietus-Snyder, M., Valente, A. et al. The role of fructose in the pathogenesis of NAFLD and the metabolic syndrome. Nature Reviews: Gastroenterology and Hepatology 2010; 7:251-264.

Lindqvist, A., Baelemans, A., Erlanson-Albersson, C. Effects of sucrose, glucose, and fructose on peripheral and central appetite signals. Regulatory Peptides 2008; 150: 26-32.

Loesche, W. Dental Caries and Periodontitis: Contrasting two infections that have medical implications. Infectious Disease Clinics of North America 2007; 21: 471-502.

Ludwig, D.S., Peterson, K.E., Gortmaker, S.L. Relation between consumption of sugar-sweetened drinks and childhood obesity: A prospective, observational analysis. Lancet 2001; 357: 505-8.

Lyons, J.J., Lyons, M.F., Meckler, K.A. A novel therapy for non-alcoholic steatohepatitis: essential fatty acids and urosodiol. American Journal of Gastroenterology 2007: 101:s160.

Lyons, M.F. 42 Days to a New Life: The Importance of a Balanced Fat Intake That Will Change Your Health (From Alpha to Omega). Xulon Press, 2007.

Mayes, P.A. Intermediary metabolism of fructose. American Journal of Clinical Nutrition 1993; 58: 754S-765S.

McGuinness, O.P., Cherrington, A.D. Effects of fructose on hepatic glucose metabolism. Current Opinion in Clinical Nutrition and Metabolic Care 2003; 6: 441-48.

Melanson, K.J. High-fructose corn syrup, energy intake, and appetite Regulation. American Journal of Clinical Nutritition 2008; 88:1738S-44S.

Miller, A., Adeli, K. Dietary fructose and the metabolic syndrome. Current Opinion in Gastroenterology 2008; 24: 204-209.

Miller, C.C., Martin, R.J., Whitney, M.L., et al. Intracerebroventricular injection of fructose stimulates feeding in rats. Nutritional Neuroscience 2002; 5: 359-62.

Montonen, J., Jarvinen, R., Knekt, P., et al. Consumption of sweetened beverages and intakes of fructose and glucose predict type 2 diabetes occurrence. Journal of Nutrition 2007; 137: 1447-54.

Nakagawa, T., Hu, H., Zharikov, S., et al. A causal role for uric acid in fructose-induced metabolic syndrome. American Journal of Physiology. Renal Physiology 2006; 290: F625-F31.

Nakagawa, T., Tuttle, K.R., Short, K.R., et al. Hypothesis: Fructose-induced hyperuricemia as a causal mechanism for the epidemic of the metabolic syndrome. Nature Clinical Practice Nephrology 2005; 1: 80-86.

Nguyen, S., Choi, H.K., Lustig, R.H., et al. Sugar-sweetened beverages, serum uric acid, and blood pressure in adolescents. Journal of Pediatrics 2009; 154: 807-13.

Ostos, M.A., Recaide, D., Baroukh, N., et al. Fructose intake increases hyperlipidemia and modifies apolipoprotein expression in apolipoprotein AI-CIII-AIV transgenic mice. Journal of Nutrition 2002; 132: 918-23.

Ouyang, X., Cirillo, P., Sautin, Y, et al. Fructose consumption as a risk factor for non-alcoholic fatty liver disease. Journal of Hepatology 2008; 48: 993-99.

Park, O.J., Cesar, D., Faix, D., et al. Mechanisms of fructose-induced hypertriglyceridemia in the rat. Activation of hepatic pyruvate dehydrogenase through inhibition of pyruvate dehydrogenase kinase. Biochemical Journal 1992; 282: 753-57.

Parks, E.J., Hellerstein, M.K. Carbohydrate-Induced Hypertriacylglycerolemia: Historical perspective and review of biological mechanisms. American Journal of Clinical Nutrition 2000; 71: 412-33.

Perez-Pozo, S.E., Schold, J., Nakagawa, T., et al. Excessive fructose intake induces the features of metabolic syndrome in healthy adult men: Role of uric acid in the hypertensive response. International Journal of Obesity 2010; 34: 454-61.

Perman, J.A. Digestion and absorption of fruit juice carbohydrates. Journal of the American College of Nutrition 1996; 15: S12-S17.

Ravich, W.J., Bayless, T.M., Thomas, M. Fructose: Incomplete intestinal absorption in humans. Gastroenterology 1983; 84: 26-29.

Ravnskov, Uffe. The Cholesterol Myths: Exposing the fallacy that saturated fat and cholesterol cause heart disease. New Trends Publishing, 2000.

Riby, J.E., Takuji, F., Dretchmer, N. Fructose absorption. American Journal of Clinical Nutrition 1993; 58: S748-S53.

Romero-Corral, A., Montori, V.M., Somers, V.K., et al. Association of bodyweight with total mortality and with cardiovascular events in coronary artery disease: A systematic review of cohort studies. Lancet 2006; 19;368(9536):666-78.

Romero-Corral, A., Somers, V.K., Sierra-Johnson, J., et al. Accuracy of body mass index in diagnosing obesity in the adult general population. International Journal of Obesity 2008; 32:959-65.

Rumessen, J.J. Fructose and food related carbohydrates. Sources, intake, absorption, and clinical implications. Scandinavian Journal of Gastroenterology 1992; 27: 819-28.

Rumessen, J.J., Gudmand-Hoyer, E. Absorption capacity of fructose in healthy adults. Comparison with sucrose and its constituent monosaccharides. Gut 1986; 27: 1161-68.

Rumessen, J.J., Gudmand-Hoyer, E. Functional bowel disease: Malabsorption and abdominal distress after ingestion of fructose, sorbitol, and fructose-sorbitol mixtures. Gastroenterology 1988; 95: 694-700.

Sabate, J.M. et al. High prevalence of small intestinal bacterial overgrowth in patients with morbid obesity:

a contributor to severe hepatic steatosis. Obesity Surgery 2008; 18: 371-77.

Sanchez-Lozada, L.G., Mu, W., Roncal, C., et al. Comparison of free fructose and glucose to sucrose in the ability to cause fatty liver. European Journal of Nutrition 2010; 49:1-9.

Sanchez-Lozada, L.G., Tapia, E., Bautista-Garcia, P., et al. Effects of febuxostat on metabolic and renal alterations in rats with fructose-induced metabolic syndrome. American Journal of Physiology (Renal Physiology) 2008; 294: F710-F718.

Skoog, S.M., Bharucha, A.E. Dietary fructose and gastrointestinal symptoms: A Review. American Journal of Gastroenterology 2004; 99: 2046-50.

Schretlen, D.J., Inscore, A.B., Vannorsdall, T.D., et al. Serum uric acid and brain ischemia in normal elderly adults. Neurology 2007; 69: 1418-23.

Schulze, M.B., Manson, J.E., Ludwig, D.S., et al. Sugar-sweetened beverages, weight gain, and incidence of type 2 diabetes in young and middle-aged women. Journal of the American Medical Association 2004; 292: 927-34.

Segal, M.S., Gollub, E., Johnson, R.J. Is the fructose index more relevant with regards to cardiovascular disease than the glycemic index? European Journal of Nutrition 2007; 46: 406-17.

Shepherd, S.J., Gibson, P.R. Fructose malabsorption and symptoms of irritable bowel syndrome: Guidelines for effective dietary management. Journal of the American Dietetic Association 2006; 106: 1631-39.

Songer, T.J. The Economic costs of NIDDM. Diabetes/Metabolism Reviews 1992; 8: 389-404.

Southgate, D.A.T. Digestion and metabolism of sugars. American Journal of Clinical Nutrition 1995; 62: S203-S211.

Spruss, A., Bergheim, I. Dietary fructose and intestinal barrier: potential risk factor in the pathogenesis of nonalcoholic fatty liver disease. Journal of Nutrition and Biochemistry 2009; 20: 657-662.

Stanhope, K.L., Griffen, S.C., Bair, B.R., et al. Twenty-four-hour endocrine and metabolic profiles following consumption of high-fructose corn syrup-, sucrose-, fructose-, and glucose-sweetened beverages with meals. American Journal of Clinical Nutrition 2008; 87: 1194-1203.

Stanhope, K.L., Schwarz, J.M., Keim, N.L., et al. Consuming fructose-sweetened, not glucose-sweetened, beverages increases visceral adiposity and lipids and decreases insulin sensitivity in overweight/obese humans. Journal of Clinical Investigation 2009; 119: 1322-34.

Striegel-Moore, R.H., Thompson, D., Affenito, S.G., et al. Correlates of beverage intake in adolescent girls: The national heart, lung and blood institute growth and health study. Journal of Pediatrics 2006; 148: 183-87.

Stirpe, F, Della Corte, E., Bonetti E., et al. Fructose-induced hyperuricemia. Lancet 2 1970; 1310-1.

Teff, K.L., Elliott, S.S., Tschop, M. et al. Dietary fructose reduces circulating insulin and leptin, attenuates postprandial suppression of ghrelin, and increases triglycerides in women. Journal of Clinical Endocrinology and Metabolism 2004; 89: 2963-72.

Teff, K.L., Grudziak, J., Townsend, R.R., et al. Endocrine and metabolic effects of consuming fructose- and glucose-sweetened beverages with meals in obese men and women: Influence of insulin resistance on plasma triglyceride responses. Journal of Clinical Endocrinology and Metabolism 2009; 94: 1562-69.

Thornburn, A.W., Storlien, L.H., Jenkins, A.B., et al. Fructose-induced in vivo insulin resistance and elevated plasma triglyceride levels in rats. American Journal of Clinical Nutrition 1989; 49: 1155-63.

Thuy, S., et al. Nonalcoholic fatty liver disease in humans is associated with increased plasma endotoxin and plasminogen activator inhibitor-1 concentrations and with fructose intake. Journal of Nutrition 2008; 138:1452-1455.

Tordoff, M., Alleva, A.M. Effect of drinking soda sweetened with aspartame or high-fructose corn syrup on food intake and body weight. American Journal of Clinical Nutrition 1990; 51: 963-69.

Truswell, A.S., Seach, J.M., Thorburn, A.W. Incomplete absorption of pure fructose in healthy subjects and the facilitating effect of glucose. American Journal of Clinical Nutrition 1988; 48: 1424-30.

Valente, A., Mietus-Snyder, M.L., Lim, J.S. et al. Association between sugar sweetened beverage consumption and serum alanine aminotransferase in obese children. Pediatric Academic Society 2009; 3854.45 [abstract].

Warner, M.L., Harley, K., Bradman, A., et al. Soda consumption and overweight status of 2 year old Mexican American children in California. Obesity 2006; 14:1966-1974.

Weiss, R., Dziura, J., Burgert, T.S., et al. Obesity and the metabolic syndrome in children and adolescents. New England Journal of Medicine 2004; 350: 2362-74.

Wheeler, M.L., Pi-Sunyer, F.X. Carbohydrate Issues: Type and amount. Journel of the American Dietetic Association 2008; 108: S34-9.

Wu, T., Giovannucci, E., Pischon, T., et al. Fructose, glycemic load, and quantity and quality of carbohydrate in relation to plasma C-peptide concentrations in

U.S. women. American Journal of Clinical Nutrition 2004; 80: 1043-49.

www.acg.org/qualityandscience/clinical/bethesda/beth30/ jac1127b.htm. 30th Bethesda Conference: The Future of Academic Cardiology.

www.cdc.gov/nchs/fastats/deaths.html. Death and Mortality from the Centers for Disease Control and Prevention.

www.ers.usda.gov/Publications/SSS/Aug05/SSS/24301. Sweetener consumption in the United States: Distribution by demographic and product character-istics. By Haley, S., et al.

www.fda.gov/bbs/topics/CONSUMER/CON00133.html. Not Only Sugar is Sweet, by Alexandra Greeley.

www.letsmove.gov. White House Task Force on Childhood Obesity Report to the President: Solving the Problem of Childhood Obesity within a Generation.

www.spc.noaa.gov/faq/tornado/killers.html. The 25 dead-liest U.S. Tornadoes.

www.USGS.gov/newsroom. Statistics Concerning Earthquakes.

www.findarticles.com/p/articles/mi_m0eub/is_1_13/ai_ 78166941. Current Knowledge of the Health Effects of Sugar Intake, by Anne L. Mardis.

Zimmet, P., Alberti, K.G., Shaw, J. Global and Societal Implications of the Diabetes Epidemic. Nature 2001; 414: 782-87.

Index of Tables